Praise for *Reboot Your Health*

'A remarkable compilation for today – updating age-old principles of holistic medicine inherited from our forefathers across the centuries from previous civilizations. I learned quite a lot about myself...'

HARVEY WHITE DM, MCH, FRCS, EMERITUS SURGEON, ROYAL MARSDEN HOSPITAL

'The key to the future of medicine is to make people more responsible for their own health. Most symptoms are due to minor alterations in the intricate balance of the human body. The advice given here is your personal trainer to make you feel better in yourself.'

PROFESSOR KAROL SIKORA, LEADING ONCOLOGIST AND DEAN OF THE UNIVERSITY OF BUCKINGHAM MEDICAL SCHOOL, FORMER HEAD OF THE WORLD HEALTH ORGANIZATION

'This book educates and underpins your good health. The only way for true preventative or anti-ageing medicine is to map your vital signs over a period of time and see where there is a trend beginning. This book instructs you how to measure these signs and what to do about it. Well done Sara!'

JOHN OGDEN DNM

'Sara Davenport has done us all a great service, in the same way that she has helped so many thousands of women through her passion for breast cancer care. Read this, do what she says and be better for it.'

P.T. BROWN PHD, FACULTY PROFESSOR FOR ORGANISATIONAL NEUROSCIENCE, MONARCH BUSINESS SCHOOL, SWITZERLAND

REBOOT

your

Health

REBOOT
your
Health

SIMPLE DIY TESTS AND SOLUTIONS TO ASSESS AND IMPROVE YOUR HEALTH

SARA DAVENPORT

HAY HOUSE

Carlsbad, California • New York City
London • Sydney • New Delhi

Published in the United Kingdom by:
Hay House UK Ltd, Astley House, 33 Notting Hill Gate, London W11 3JQ
Tel: +44 (0)20 3675 2450; Fax: +44 (0)20 3675 2451
www.hayhouse.co.uk

Published in the United States of America by:
Hay House Inc., PO Box 5100, Carlsbad, CA 92018-5100
Tel: (1) 760 431 7695 or (800) 654 5126
Fax: (1) 760 431 6948 or (800) 650 5115
www.hayhouse.com

Published in Australia by:
Hay House Australia Ltd, 18/36 Ralph St, Alexandria NSW 2015
Tel: (61) 2 9669 4299; Fax: (61) 2 9669 4144
www.hayhouse.com.au

Published in India by:
Hay House Publishers India, Muskaan Complex,
Plot No.3, B-2, Vasant Kunj, New Delhi 110 070
Tel: (91) 11 4176 1620; Fax: (91) 11 4176 1630
www.hayhouse.co.in

A catalogue record for this book is available from the British Library.

ISBN: 978-1-78817-055-0

Interior illustrations by Liron Gilenberg | www.ironicitalics.com

Printed and bound by CPI Group (UK) Ltd, Croydon, CR0 4YY

For Alnur, with all my love.

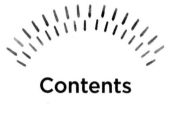

Contents

Contents

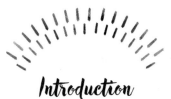

Introduction

Why Settle for Poor Health?

'Take care of your body. It's the only place you have to live.'

JIM ROHN

Close your eyes and sit quietly for a moment. Tune into your body... How are you feeling?

Do you feel energized? Or tired? Do your muscles, joints and, as far as you can sense them, internal organs feel relaxed and well, or tense and sluggish? Have you forgotten how you used to feel when you were younger? When you leaped out of bed full of enthusiasm, went to the gym for hours, could walk 5km (3 miles) with no problems, garden for hours on end and stay up all night partying before doing a full day of work the next day? Has that energy disappeared or seeped away without you realizing?

Perhaps you've visited your doctor for a particular issue, hoping for a diagnosis, and tried a range of different therapies and medications. You may have learned to live with your symptoms, resigning yourself to the idea that you will always feel this way.

But you really don't need to settle for poor health. In order to work out what is causing your problems you simply need to examine every aspect of your life so that you can work out what has made you unwell.

Think of it like gardening...

Imagine that you have a beautiful garden and in it there is a rare and special plant: it lives in a pot and has bloomed there happily, year after year. But one day you notice that it is looking sick.

Imagine what you would do. You would look carefully at every aspect of the situation to find out what was the matter, and then take whatever steps were necessary to get it flourishing again. You would check to see if the plant had become rootbound and whether it needs repotting. You would look for signs of fungus on its leaves. You might test the soil and notice that the earth around the plant lacks nutrients and needs fertilizer. You would remove any weeds and garden pests, and water it thoroughly, confident in the knowledge that each one of your actions would help it flourish again.

Exactly the same is true for you. If, like that plant, you are low in energy or in poor health, you need to take similar steps to restore yourself to vibrant wellbeing. Together with your doctor, this book can help you to undertake a thorough analysis of your health. Once you have a comprehensive picture you can then take whatever decisions are necessary to restore balance and usher in a healthier, happier you.

All health issues have specific roots and it is my belief, having worked with hundreds of clients, that stress is the hidden cause in most cases.[1] You may not even be fully aware of how stress affects you. It might not necessarily be what's happening in your life that's causing your problems, but simply that your lifestyle is putting your physical body under duress. But whatever your symptoms, the treatment needs to be specifically tailored to you and, in order to prevent further problems, the underlying stresses need to be identified and dealt with too.

In the following chapters, you'll find a holistic blueprint for wellbeing – a manual for good health that you can follow from this day forwards. It will help you to get a clear and detailed map of your health, drawing on the wisdom of a wide range of tests, questionnaires, therapies and techniques. There are a variety of suggestions for how to resolve any issues and restore yourself to good health, simply and inexpensively.

Creating wellness

I have spent almost 20 years working with people diagnosed with cancer, many of whom have now recovered. I have observed, in the choices they have made, what seems to work well for the vast majority of people.

In 1997, I set up a cancer charity, Breast Cancer Haven, which offers support, counselling and complementary therapies to anyone, anywhere, affected by breast cancer, entirely free of charge. Our first centre opened in Fulham, London in 2000. Since then, we have opened further centres in Hereford, Leeds, Worcester, Hampshire and Solihull. Breast Cancer Haven is now one of the UK's leading national breast cancer charities and has delivered hundreds of thousands of free treatments to tens of thousands of people. The average visitor makes repeat visits, over a period of months. We don't offer a quick fix, but our visitors tell us that the therapy and support we offer is life changing.

Although Breast Cancer Haven is a breast cancer charity, through my work I've developed passion and knowledge about all aspects of health and wellbeing. I've met with a huge range of practitioners and therapists, and observed diverse approaches in action. As part of this process, I've developed a deep understanding of the insidious nature of hidden stress, and the powerful, varied and, often, unlikely ways to treat it. I've been surprised, impressed and excited by a wide range of diagnostic techniques and therapies, and in my blog (reboothealth.co.uk) I look at many of these topics in greater depth. Not all of them have the backing of conventional medical science and some have been criticized both in the press and by scientists, but I believe it's worth keeping an open mind and listening to anecdotal evidence, rather than being limited by more rigid conventional medical practice.

We live in a culture where we're conditioned to hand over all our power and autonomy to the 'experts' – whether that's our doctor or a consultant. There is some good sense in this, obviously, but deep down, all of us are aware that many of these experts have views that are subjective, generalist and unquestionably constrained by extreme time pressure, financial considerations and the limited range of treatments available to them.

Your body whispers before it shouts™

So much of your wellbeing is in your hands. In many instances, there really is no need to wait for somebody else to make you feel better.

But this means taking responsibility for your wellbeing by tuning into your body, looking at your symptoms and examining your surroundings because, like the plant metaphor I gave earlier, poor health doesn't manifest randomly. It rarely appears out of the blue. Your body has probably been sending you signals for some time: asking for attention, providing clues.

In our super-busy world, however, overwhelmed by the noise of life, with the shouty demands of work and jam-packed family and social lives, it takes a special sort of discipline and awareness to hear your body's whispers. Our attention is constantly under siege, with the incessant pinging of gadgets, expectations of immediate response and the deeply distracting sense that we're all living life on multiple platforms, all of which require us to service them constantly. It's exhausting and trains us to always be hovering at the edge of the moment, thinking about the next thing, or what we haven't done, rather than what is going on NOW. Make the conscious decision to pay your body and mind the deep attention they've been crying out for, and start acting to redress the balance, and you'll feel a difference in your wellbeing, quickly. After only three weeks, I guarantee you'll notice a marked improvement.

The various exploratory tests and wide range of treatment suggestions – therapeutic, dietary, emotional and psychological – aim to help you to better understand, as well as heal, your body and mind. Rather than a rushed five-minute window for discussion, diagnosis and prescription, you'll have the time you need to explore, understand, investigate and research the right solutions. I say solutions because there will be more than one hidden stressor at work and in order to tackle whatever yours turn out to be, you're likely to need to adopt a holistic approach to restore the balance.

TOP TIP

Many of us blame the state of our body and mind on our ancestry or genes. But only a quarter of the state of your health is down to genetics, the rest is down to lifestyle and stress management.[2] Lifestyle changes can definitely improve your health. It's never too late to make them – even if you are in your older years.

Using this book

There are three simple steps to a life of good health and this book is designed to help you to:

1. Understand where you are now.

2. Rebalance your body and mind.

3. Monitor your wellbeing in the future.

The best person to take on this task is the person who knows every aspect of your life inside out: YOU. You have to become your own health detective and learn to read the clues your body and mind is sending you. Once you have decoded these, you will have the answers you need to heal yourself.

In Part I, we'll look specifically at the body and each of its major organs and systems in turn. Take each of the simple tests in every chapter and work through them, one by one. Most of the tests are simple, inexpensive and, most importantly, have no side-effects, while others will require you to visit a health professional. Those marked with this ⌂ symbol can either be done at home or online. Others marked by the ✚ symbol can be accessed via your doctor, nutritionist or other health professional. You'll also find some simple remedies and practices, shown with this 🌱 symbol, which you can use to help support or alleviate health issues.

TOP TIP

I strongly recommend running all of the tests to get a truly in-depth view of your health. It's important to be thorough and test every one of them to establish what's up.

In Part II, we'll look at lifestyle, your nutrition, exercise, sleeping patterns and environment, as well as the mind and the role of stress.

In every chapter, you'll find simple actions that you can take to restore the balance of your wellbeing. Often, we are out of balance on a number of levels and a combination of things is likely to be contributing to your symptoms. Take your time and don't expect to solve this puzzle instantly.

TOP TIP

Before starting out, you might like to buy a notebook to record your health results and observations. Write down the date you run each test and what action you decide to take, and then you will be able to track your progress clearly.

An overview before you start

I'd like you to start by examining how your energy, happiness and health feel right now.

ENERGY SCAN

 Home

Just like a car, you are powered by energy 'batteries', so take a moment to tune into your energy levels.

1. Sit quietly somewhere and really listen to how your body is feeling.

2. Imagine that there is a battery inside you – a store of energy – powering your body and marked with the numbers 1–10 at regular intervals from bottom to top.

3. On that 1–10 scale, how full is your battery?

4. Write down the number that instantly springs into your mind, along with the date.

5. You can refer back to it in a few weeks' time when you've had a chance to introduce some of the rebalancing suggestions in this book. Then retest again and compare the results.

In our frenetic modern lives, we're often running so fast that it's not just our physical body we neglect; we hardly have time to notice what is going on in the rest of our lives either. Did you fulfil your earlier hopes and dreams, or drift along until you found yourself somewhere else entirely? Have you been climbing a ladder and now, having reached the top, found you placed it against the wrong wall?

LIFE SCAN

 Home

We rarely, if ever, take the time to stop, look at where we are going and decide if that's the direction we really want to travel in for the rest of our lives. Take that time now.

Using the 1–10 scale, where 10 is 'as good as it could get' and 1 is 'terrible', take a moment to answer the following questions:

- How does your life feel overall now?

- How much do you like your job?

- How much do you like your home?

- How are your relationships? (Rate each of your relationships: parents, partner, children, work colleagues, etc.)

- Do you have enough time for yourself?

- How many hours a week do you spend with friends having fun?

- How much time do you spend helping others?

HAPPINESS SCAN

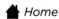 *Home*

Next, become conscious of how happy you feel. Are you happy? Or have you been hiding from yourself for years? If you don't even realize that you're unhappy then you're never likely to make the changes that will get you to a happier place.

1. Sit down somewhere quiet, with your eyes shut, and just breathe deeply for a few minutes.

2. Now really notice how you feel. Simply let the day-to-day stuff go and let any fears, worries or difficult people or situations, which you may have been blocking out, flood through you.

3. Then on a scale of 1 to 10, where 1 is 'everything is fine' and 10 is 'it couldn't get any worse', rate how happy you are right here and now.

4. Don't try to make it better or worse than it actually is. It may even feel 20/10 bad – that's fine. Just find the number and write it down.

BODY SCAN

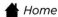 *Home*

Next up, I'd like you to consider your physical health.

1. List any physical symptoms that are worrying you.

2. List any diagnosed issues, along with any medication you are taking and the dosage.

3. What's your current weight?

4. On average, how many times a week do you currently exercise?

5. On average, how many hours do you sleep each night? And how many times do you wake up at night?

6. Close your eyes and, on a scale of 1-10, write down the single number that comes into your head that represents how well you currently feel physically.

These four tests will give you a baseline to which you can refer over the months and years to come. Down the line it is often hard to remember how well you were, or how you felt, before you started on your health journey.

If you feel you have a lot to uncover and restore, please don't worry, as creating a healthier, happier you is a step-by-step process. Each change that you make will move you closer to your goal. Set your intentions clearly and, in a remarkably short period of time, you'll find that you arrive at where you want to go.

Your health is in your hands. It's entirely up to you.

Part 1

Body Basics

'It does not matter how slowly you go as long as you do not stop.'

CONFUCIUS

Chapter 1

The Heart:
Your Life Force

'The heart is our strongest muscle; like any muscle, the heart grows stronger with use.'

DAN MILLMAN

Your heart sits in your chest between your lungs, slightly to the left of your breastbone. It has four chambers and is approximately the same size as a fist. It beats more than 100,000 times a day, pumping about 1,000 litres (265 gallons) of blood around the body, and is the only organ in the body that isn't susceptible to cancer.

However, coronary heart disease (CHD) affects one in every three families worldwide and kills more people in the UK and across the globe than any other disease.[1] CHD is the result of a process called 'atherosclerosis', the build-up of fatty deposits on the walls of the arteries around the heart, which restricts the flow of blood to the heart muscle and can lead to serious health issues.

The following increases your risk of stroke and CHD:[2]

- Smoking

- High blood pressure (hypertension)

- High cholesterol levels: Cholesterol is a fat made naturally by your body, mainly in the liver. It is needed to keep your cells healthy, and latest research at the time of writing indicates that elevated levels are a result not of poor diet but excessive inflammation, which can endanger your health.

- Not taking regular exercise

- Diabetes

- Being overweight

- Having a family history of CHD

Stress is also an issue, although medical research hasn't proved exactly how it increases the risk of heart disease. It may be that stress increases other risk factors (such as weight gain or high blood pressure) or that we respond to it by making unhealthy lifestyle choices, such as drinking too much alcohol or caffeine, overeating, smoking or not exercising. We do know that chronic stress exposes the body to persistently elevated blood pressure and elevated levels of stress hormones like adrenaline and cortisol, which can lead to inflammation and so increase the risk of blood clots and heart attack.[3]

Heart-wise

There are three different measurements to look at when checking your heart:

- Blood pressure

- Heart rate

- Cholesterol and triglyceride levels

The first two tests you can do at home and your doctor can do the third. They are also available in some pharmacies.

BLOOD PRESSURE TEST

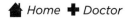 Home ✚ *Doctor*

You can measure your blood pressure by using an electronic blood pressure machine – an inflatable cuff attached to a monitor that gives a digital readout of your blood pressure and pulse. If you want to take regular readings, you can buy a monitor or make regular visits to your pharmacy or doctor.

Always take your blood pressure readings twice. First, note your pulse (see page 23) when you are seated and relaxed. Then stand up and test again. The exertion should cause your blood pressure to increase and your resting pulse rate to go up. If your blood pressure drops when you stand up, this may indicate adrenal fatigue (see also Chapter 13, page 110). Book an appointment with your doctor for a check-up and treatment options.

Understanding your results

The reading will consist of two numbers, i.e. 110/80.

The first number is your systolic blood pressure level. When your heart beats, it contracts, pushing blood through your arteries creating pressure. A normal reading is 120 or below; 120–139 is normal but higher than the ideal and indicates a slightly elevated risk of developing heart disease; 140 or higher, in repeated measurements, is high blood pressure.

The second number is the diastolic blood pressure level and indicates the pressure in the arteries when your heart rests between beats. A normal reading is 80 or less; 80–89 is higher than ideal; 90 or higher, in repeated measurements, is indicative of high blood pressure.

If you're diagnosed with high blood pressure, your doctor may recommend medication in order to reduce your risk of developing heart disease.

A reading of less than 90/60 is low blood pressure.

High blood pressure (hypertension)

Called 'the silent killer' because it catches so many people unawares, high blood pressure puts strain on your heart and blood vessels, and so increases your risk of heart attack and stroke. It can also lead to heart and kidney disease, and is closely linked to some forms of dementia. Plaque deposits may be clogging up your blood flow, and this can eventually lead to clots and ultimately a stroke.

Action plan

→ **Don't smoke:** Visit your local pharmacy or doctor and make a plan to stop. Most health authorities run smoke-free campaigns and can offer one-to-one support and advice to help you quit.

→ **Cut down alcohol:** Heavy drinking (defined as more than 4 units per day for men and 3 units for women per day) can lead to an increased risk of high blood pressure, so make sure you stay within the advised limits.

→ **Maintain a healthy weight:** Moderate exercise for 30 minutes or more, five times a week can help lower your blood pressure, reduce inflammation and improve your cholesterol levels.[4] (See also Chapter 21.)

TOP TIP

Physical activity will temporarily cause your blood pressure to rise whilst you are exercising and return to normal as soon as you stop. So, if you have high blood pressure readings, it's always a good idea to check with your doctor before starting any new exercise regime.

➔ **Keep caffeine to a minimum:** Caffeine can temporarily raise your heart rate and blood pressure. If you regularly have more than four cups of coffee a day, it's a good idea to start cutting down.[5] Substitute coffee with green tea, which is packed full of antioxidants, or caffeine-free rooibos tea. Herbal teas, hot lemon water or just plain filtered water are other healthy alternatives.

➔ **Cut down salt:** Salt increases the amount of sodium in your bloodstream, which then overloads your kidneys and can result in water retention, higher blood pressure and bloating. The good news is that if you reduce your salt (to no more than 1 teaspoon a day), your blood pressure readings will improve within a month.[6]

➔ **Supplement:** Add in the following foods and/or supplements where you can:

- Vitamin C reduces triglycerides and cholesterol levels (see also page 27), repairs and regenerates tissues, strengthens blood vessels and helps keep your arteries soft.[7] The recommended daily dosage is 100mg a day, but upping it to 400mg a day will keep your energy levels high and any excess that your body doesn't need will be excreted in your urine. For an additional boost eat more vitamin C rich fruits and vegetables: red pepper, citrus fruits, kiwi, broccoli and Brussels sprouts all contain high levels.

~ There is a strong connection between heart attack risk and magnesium deficiency.[8] Legumes (e.g. lentils, chickpeas, etc.), nuts, green leafy vegetables and wholegrains (e.g. brown rice and wholegrain bread) will boost your magnesium levels, which should ideally be 1.7–2.2mg/dL (0.7–0.91mmol/L.) If using a supplement, take 600mg a day as a minimum.

~ Add healthy oils to your diet by including omega-3 flaxseed oil or eating two to three portions of oily fish each week (e.g. sardines, mackerel, salmon or trout). These heart-healthy oils have been shown to lower blood pressure, ease inflammation and repair arteries.[9]

~ CoQ10 has been shown to reduce blood pressure by 9 per cent when 100mg is taken twice daily over 12 weeks.[10]

~ A daily combination of B vitamins, including B6 (40mg daily), B12 (200mcg daily) and folic acid (800mcg), has been shown to reduce high blood pressure in women[11] by 46 per cent.

➜ **Manage stress:** Anxiety and trauma can make your heart beat faster, bringing on panic attacks and heart fluttering, raising your blood pressure and narrowing your blood vessels, so avoid stress or find ways of managing it. (See also Chapter 22.)

➜ **Drink organic olive leaf tea:** Caffeine- and tannin-free, this tea can help regulate blood pressure by decreasing arterial stiffness;[12] it is also four times higher in antioxidants than green tea, as well as having antibiotic, antiviral and antifungal properties. Amazingly, it actually tastes nice, too.

→ **Try a cup of beetroot juice:** Drinking 1 cup of beetroot juice a day for a week can improve blood flow, as it contains high levels of nitrates, which cause your blood vessels to dilate and so lowers your blood pressure. Contraindicated for anyone diagnosed with diabetes.[13]

Low blood pressure (hypotension)

Low blood pressure means that your heart is not pushing out your blood with sufficient strength so your tissues and organs won't receive enough oxygen and nutrients. Low blood pressure can also indicate that your adrenals and thyroid are struggling (see also Chapters 12–13). Some people have naturally low blood pressure, which doesn't need to be treated, but if your blood pressure readings are low and you regularly feel faint, dizzy or shaky (particularly after missing a meal), then make an appointment with your doctor for a check-up.

Action plan

→ **Manage your salt intake:** Not eating enough salt can be as bad as eating too much, so ensure that you're eating some (no more than 1 teaspoon) each day and include some salty foods (e.g. olives or seaweed) if necessary.

→ **Drink water:** Drink at least 1.5 litres (3 pints) of water a day, as dehydration can lower your blood pressure.

→ **Supplement:**

~ If you have coeliac disease or an alcohol problem, you may not be absorbing folic acid efficiently and this can cause low blood pressure.[14] Certain medications also deplete folic acid so consult your doctor for advice. Supplement with 400mg daily and increase your consumption of leafy green vegetables, asparagus, beans, nuts and liver.

~ Low vitamin B12 levels can result in anaemia and trigger low blood pressure.[15] Ensure you're getting enough B12 in your diet (e.g. eggs, dairy, chicken, fish and beef) and/ or supplementing daily with 1,000–3,000mcg.

~ Bee pollen contains rutin, which strengthens blood vessels and lowers cholesterol. It has anti-clotting mechanisms that protect against stroke and heart attack. Take one to two tablespoons of raw granules or three 500mg capsules daily. (See also Chapters 12–13.)

~ Taking 500–3,000mg daily of Siberian ginseng (dried root as a tea or capsule or half to one teaspoon of tincture two to three times a day) has been shown to raise low blood pressure levels effectively.[16]

~ Liquorice root can also raise low blood pressure levels.[17] Drink it as a tea or in capsule form. This is a powerful natural remedy so the dosage needs to be tailored to your requirements by a nutritional practitioner or naturopath, who can also monitor your improvement.

➔ **Eat smaller meals:** Your body needs large amounts of energy to digest large meals and this can cause blood pressure fluctuations, so make your mantra 'eat little and often'.

➔ **Get a boost:** Drinking two cups of coffee in the morning can increase your blood pressure.

TOP TIP

Blood Pressure Companion is a free app that tracks your numbers. But if you want more precise measurements then invest in a QardioArm, a smart blood pressure monitor that accurately measures, records and tracks your results.

HEART RATE TEST

 Home

Your heart rate is an indicator of your overall fitness level and heart health. For an accurate reading, take this test soon after rising in the morning, by finding your pulse either on your wrist or neck:

1. Using the middle and index fingers of one hand, press them firmly on the artery on the inside of the wrist of your other hand or into the soft hollow to the side of your windpipe, until you can clearly feel your pulse.

2. Count how many beats in a minute (or 20 seconds and then multiply by three).

3. Repeat the test three times to get an average score of your resting heart rate.

Understanding your results

A normal reading will be between 60 and 80 beats per minute (bpm). The more your body is struggling with stress, weight, lack of exercise, medications and/or emotional difficulties, the greater the strain on your heart and the higher your reading.

Low heart rate (bradycardia)

Less than 60bpm counts as a slow heart rate and whether this is a problem or not depends on your age and fitness. A low heart rate is usually considered healthy if you are superfit, but it also reduces the amount of oxygen being pumped around your body and, if you are not in peak condition, can leave you – and your organs – exhausted. The heart muscles weaken as we age and so your numbers may drop, indicating potential health issues and a problem with the heart's electrical system.

Hypothyroidism can affect your heart rate, as can medications (i.e. beta-blockers) specifically designed to bring your heart rate down. Different temperatures, stress and certain foods can also affect your numbers, as can sleep apnoea.

It is important to establish your personal baseline and record your pulse readings two or three times a week over a period of a few months. If you regularly have a reading of less than 55–60bpm, book a check-up with your doctor, who may do an ECG (electrocardiogram) and can advise you how to treat any issues or refer you to a specialist for further advice. The same advice applies if your pulse is continuously rapid with readings over 120bpm or if there is a sudden and sustained change to your baseline readings.

Action plan

→ **Try meditation and yoga:** Both of these practices have been shown to reduce arrhythmia and bring the heart rate back to normal.[18]

→ **Get some rest:** Low oxygenation in the blood may mean you struggle to sleep and lack energy during the day. (See also Chapter 23.)

➜ **Breathe:** Deep breathing exercises will increase the oxygen levels in your blood (see Chapter 22, page 212).

➜ **Avoid alcohol:** Don't drink more than three to four units of alcohol a day because it dilates the blood vessels, lowering blood pressure levels further. Moderate drinking is thought to be safe for most people with bradycardia. Always check with your doctor.

➜ **Get to a healthy weight:** Review your weight and diet to reduce the pressure on your heart. (See also Chapters 17 and 19.)

➜ **Book in for acupuncture:** Shown to bring low heart rates back to normal[19] by calming a rapid heart rate, acupuncture can also boost a weak pulse and poor circulation. Book in for regular sessions and monitor any changes.

TOP TIP

Kardia is a phone app that analyses your heart signals and rhythms, comparing them to its internal database to diagnose arrhythmia and vascular problems. An incredible 90 per cent of strokes could be prevented by early detection of cardiac anomalies.

High heart rate (tachycardia)

See your doctor as soon as possible if your resting heart rate is over 100bpm, or you feel your heart racing, have palpitations or get stabbing pains in the chest, as it may be a sign that your heart is beating too rapidly, reducing blood flow and oxygen to the rest of your body.

REDUCE YOUR HEART RATE

🌿 Remedy

For an immediate solution to a rapid heartbeat, wrap an ice pack in a thin towel and place on your face to slow the vagal nerve that regulates your heartbeat. Be sure to seek medical advice if a rapid heart rate is a regular occurrence and/or your heart rate is more than 100bpm.

Action plan

→ **Exercise:** The heart is a muscle and the fitter it is, the less hard it has to work so exercise, exercise, exercise. You don't need to start a strenuous fitness regime in order to benefit your heart (and it is not advised if you have heart rate issues). Just 30 minutes of moderate exercise, such as walking or swimming, five times a week makes a difference and can reduce inflammation. (See also Chapter 21.)

→ **Reduce stress:** Identify and resolve stress; it affects your heart. (See also Chapter 22.)

→ **Maintain a healthy weight:** This takes the pressure off your heart. (See also Chapter 17.)

→ **Stretch:** Regular yoga or pranayama breathing practice increases blood flow and oxygenation and can help lower your heart rate.

→ **Rest:** Make sure you get quality sleep. (See also Chapter 23.)

→ **Supplement:** Eat potassium-rich foods, such as raisins, dates and bananas, as these have been shown to heal tachycardia naturally.[20]

TOP TIP

The heart rate app Cardiio monitors your pulse, collects information on your heart health, offers suggested workouts and tracks your progress. Or check out the Karvonen Heart Rate Calculator – another online solution.

Cholesterol

Cholesterol is a wax-like, fatty substance made in the liver and the small intestine and is essential for brain development. It protects your nerves from damage, improves the elasticity of your red blood cells and skin, and increases the production of both sex and stress hormones. It is vitally important for your body and is taken in and out of the arteries by tiny 'taxi' transporters, the lipoprotein carriers LDL (low-density lipoprotein) and HDL (high-density lipoprotein).

Until a few years ago, your doctor would likely tell you that the higher your HDL, the lower your risk of heart problems, and the higher your LDL, the greater. They described HDL and LDL simply but memorably for the rest of us as 'good' and 'bad' cholesterol, despite the fact that HDL and LDL are not cholesterol at all but lipoprotein carriers. High levels of LDL were said to be the result of the food you ate: an overly fatty diet and certain cholesterol 'baddies' – red meat, eggs and cheese in particular.

'Safe' levels of cholesterol have been repeatedly lowered in the UK over the last few decades, and, perhaps driven by the pharmaceutical industry's pill-pushing agenda, standard medical procedure has been to keep more and more people on statins for the rest of their lives. Side-effects include joint and muscle pain, liver damage, headaches and a whole list of other nasties, and yet research shows that you can take statins for years and still only gain an additional three days of life![21]

Today, cardiologists and up-to-date doctors take a very different approach. Recent studies have shown that there is, in fact, no evidence that connects fatty foods with high cholesterol levels, or high cholesterol levels with heart disease – or stroke or Type 2 diabetes – and no link at all to early death from high cholesterol. In fact, the reverse is true – eating more rather than less fat was found to slow atherosclerosis, and researchers found it was carbohydrate, not fat, that increased the problem. They concluded that cholesterol is a sign of chronic inflammation in the body, and that the best way to reduce this inflammation is simply by eating proper whole foods and walking briskly for half an hour every day.[22-25]

TOP TIP

For more in-depth information read Dr Zoe Harcombe's brilliant blog on cholesterol: zoeharcombe.com.

CHOLESTEROL TEST

🏠 *Home* ➕ *Doctor*

Cholesterol is currently estimated with a fasting blood test, meaning you may drink only water for 12 hours beforehand. Your doctor is the best person to test your cholesterol, but DIY kits are available over the pharmacy counter and online.

Understanding your results

Your doctor will use the following guide to understand your numbers:

LDL: Up to 3mmol/L is acceptable.

HDL: You want a number between 1.2–1.7mmol/L.

Total cholesterol: This is the overall total amount of cholesterol (HDL and LDL) and an ideal range is 4.9–5.4mmol/L. Be aware that tests are often out by up to 19 per cent.

Total cholesterol/HDL: If your HDL is high, the risk of cardiovascular problems and atherosclerosis is considered low. If your HDL is low, then it is more of a problem. A low HDL is thought to be more dangerous than high total cholesterol.

Non-HDL cholesterol: This is your total cholesterol minus your HDL. The level of your non-HDL is thought to be an even more accurate indicator of risk of cardiovascular disease than your LDL (bad) cholesterol.

TOP TIPS

- *If you're taking statins, supplement daily with 30mg CoQ10 in your body,[26] so supplement with 30mg CoQ10 daily. It supports your heart, improves the strength of your blood vessels and lowers your cholesterol levels, as well as reducing muscle aches and other statin side-effects.[27] As ever, check with your doctor before adding it to your daily supplement regime.*

- *Red yeast rice extract is a natural alternative if you find you can't tolerate statins.*

- *If you're pregnant, stressed, ill or recovering from an operation, your cholesterol levels will be higher than normal.*

Action plan

→ **Watch your fats:** Cut down on saturated fats (e.g. animal fats, full-fat dairy products and palm oil). Eat healthier fats in the form of nuts, seeds, avocados, white meats and oily fish.

→ **Eat more fibre:** Increase your intake of fruit, vegetables and wholegrains, as fibre and plant sterols bind to cholesterol and aid its excretion.

→ **Supplement:**

~ Niacin (vitamin B3) can increase your HDL by 30–35 per cent and reduce LDL by 25 per cent. Aim for 500–1,000mcg daily,[28] but buy 'no flush' niacin, because otherwise you may look as if you're constantly blushing.

~ Vitamin E helps to lower LDL cholesterol, reduces plaque build-up and may help prevent the formation of blood clots.[29-30] Optimal dosage is 400IU per day, though the average amount provided in any multivitamin supplement is likely to be around 30IU, so check the label. Foods that contain vitamin E include almonds, spinach, sweet potato, sunflower seeds and avocado.

~ Omega-3 is an important part of a heart-healthy diet and nutritionists suggest eating at least two portions of oily fish – salmon, mackerel, herring – a week. Studies have shown it reduces the risk of stroke by 50 per cent.[31]

TOP TIPS

• *Aspirin, still comes out on top as an overall cardiovascular preventative treatment.[32]*

• *Did you know that watching violent or upsetting programmes on TV for several hours at a time has been shown to drive up blood cholesterol more dramatically than your inherited genes, what you eat or a couch-potato lifestyle.[33]*

- *In the Blue Zones – the areas of the world where people regularly live happily and healthily to 110 years old – researchers have found ultra-high cholesterol levels.*

- *Eating four servings a week of nuts can reduce your risk of coronary death by 37 per cent due to their abundance of healthy oils.[34]*

Triglycerides

Although less well known than cholesterol, triglycerides are the most common type of fat in the body. They are created from the unused carbohydrate calories that you eat but don't use immediately for energy and so are stored in your fat cells for later use. Too much alcohol, fatty and sugary foods, certain prescription drugs and certain medical conditions (i.e. diabetes, kidney disease and an underactive thyroid) can all serve to increase your triglyceride levels and raise your risk of heart problems and pancreatic disease.

Abnormally low levels of triglycerides may indicate absorption or thyroid problems.[35] Slightly higher cholesterol levels, along with both higher triglycerides and TSH (thyroid-stimulating hormone), can indicate potential hypothyroidism (see Chapter 12, page 106). As a general rule, triglycerides are tested at the same time as cholesterol and if your cholesterol is high then your triglycerides are likely to be, too. Your doctor can advise the best treatment.

Chapter 2

The Lungs:
Your Breathing System

'I believe the body can take care of itself. It's all about self-health. It's about depending on our breathing.'

CARY-HIROYUKI TAGAWA

The surface area of your lungs roughly equals the size of a tennis court and they sit behind your ribs in your chest. They take in oxygen from the air when you inhale and deliver it to your blood, removing carbon dioxide and other waste products as you exhale. Your lungs also act as filters, removing dust, dirt and pollution from the air that you breathe. On average you breathe in and out 12–20 times a minute.

Did you know that the left lung is always smaller than the right and no matter how hard you try to empty your lungs, there will always be one litre (just over 2 pints) of air left?

Keep your lungs in good health now and you will reap the rewards later. Without sufficient oxygen, your tissues and organs and cells won't work properly. Poor air quality and environmental pollution can reduce your oxygen levels, so it is essential to strengthen and clear your lungs to avoid any problems at a later date. If you have breathing issues of any kind now, even the simplest steps will make a noticeable difference. And if you are a smoker, don't underestimate the effects tobacco can have on your lungs long-term.

SPIROSMART

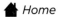 *Home*

Graduate students from the University of Washington in Seattle invented the SpiroSmart app, which you can use to measure your lung function accurately. It works by analysing your lip reverberation as you blow into your phone and assesses how much airflow is going through your trachea and vocal tract, and then compares it to healthy measurements. Ingenious.

OXYGEN LEVELS TEST

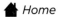 *Home*

The Nonin Go2 Finger Pulse Oximeter is an inexpensive, easy-to-use monitor that checks your oxygen saturation levels. Get an accurate reading by checking four times a day over five days (nonin.com/Home-Pulse-Oximeter). Aim for a 94–99 per cent level. Always consult your doctor for professional tests.

THE CP (CONTROL PAUSE) TEST

🏠 *Home*

This measures your body oxygen levels. Make sure you have not eaten for several hours before you do this test. Sit down and relax all your muscles for five to seven minutes. Breathe out. Pinch your nose closed and count slowly in seconds until you feel you need to take a breath. The number of seconds is the number of your score. Forty seconds or more is normal. Sixty is excellent. If your numbers are low, please consult your doctor.

Action plan

➡ **Try a herbal remedy:** Plants and herbs have been used to strengthen the lungs for centuries, but it's always best to seek advice from a qualified herbalist. Some of the best herbs to boost lung function are:

- ~ Coltsfoot tea clears excess mucus and helps with asthma, coughs and bronchitis.

- ~ Thyme treats respiratory tract infections and wipes out bacteria.

- ~ Lobelia thins mucus and breaks up congestion, clearing the airways and helping with easier breathing.

- ~ Eucalyptus contains cineole, which eases coughs and soothes irritated sinuses.

➔ **Invest in a nebulizer:** You can find more information about the benefits of use of a nebulizer at reboothealth.co.uk, but the following oils all have excellent healing properties:

~ Sage oil eases sore throats and coughs.

~ Peppermint oil contains menthol and soothes and decongests.

~ Oregano oil contains carvacrol and rosmarinic acid, both of which are decongestants and histamine reducers, boosting the respiratory tract and clearing the sinuses.

~ Liquorice root is brilliant for loosening the phlegm in the respiratory tract; it calms inflammation, expels mucus and fights off lung infections.[1]

➔ **Up your fibre:** Eat a diet rich in fruit, vegetables, beans, lentils and wholegrains to help strengthen your lungs and reduce inflammation, a factor in many lung problems.[2]

➔ **Breathe:** Breathing exercises can improve your lung capacity and boost oxygen levels in your blood. Join a yoga breathing class or use simple breathing exercises daily (see Chapter 22, page 212).

Chapter 3

The Stomach:
Your Food Processor

'All disease begins in the gut.'

HIPPOCRATES

Much of our health and wellbeing relies on the ability of the gut to digest what we eat and absorb all its goodness. Many people suffer with issues, such as bloating and IBS (irritable bowel syndrome), food intolerances or discomfort after eating.[1] Your body needs a constant source of fuel in the shape of proteins, carbohydrates, fats, vitamins and minerals, and understanding how the gut works, testing its efficiency and then righting any imbalances can often be the key to feeling well and energized.

The stomach sits in the upper left area of your tummy; this is your food processor – but a finely engineered one. It can hold around 1.5 litres (3 pints) of food and drink, and it takes about seven seconds for that food to get from your mouth to your stomach and about four hours for a moderate meal to be processed. Your stomach does this by secreting hydrochloric acid (HCL) and peptic enzymes to digest proteins, break up fibre and soften any connective tissue in foods, killing off any bugs or parasites that may have been hitching a ride in your food in the process, before delivering it to the small intestine (see Chapter 4, page 43). Everyone's stomach (as an adult) is more or less the same size – about the size of a clenched fist, whether you are tall or short, small or large. And did you know, when you blush, your stomach lining turns bright red, too?

Eating large amounts from time to time doesn't affect the size of the stomach – it will stretch to accommodate vast quantities, shrinking back to its normal size once the food has passed through your digestive tract. And however much you eat, it won't burst – though it may well feel as if it's about to! Binge daily, week after week, however, and you risk gaining a lot of excess weight and permanently stretching your stomach muscles, leaving surgery as the only option to make it smaller again.

Many stomach issues, such as heartburn and indigestion, arise from eating too quickly and can be resolved by simply slowing down at mealtimes and taking care to chew each morsel 20 times before swallowing, allowing your saliva to start breaking down the food long before it hits your stomach. If, however, you're still having the same issues after eating, then it might be time to test your stomach acid (HCL) levels. Once you have the answer, then it's always a good idea to consult your doctor for further advice and to rule out more serious issues.

LEMON JUICE TEST

 Home

Acid reflux and heartburn are more often a result of too little stomach acid (HCL) than too much.[2-3] If this is something you suffer with, the next time you have stomach pain, try taking a tablespoon of fresh lemon juice. If the pain goes away, you may have too little stomach acid. If the pain worsens then you may have too much stomach acid and possibly an ulcer, so be sure to consult your doctor.

If, and only if, your symptoms go away with the lemon juice test, follow up with the betaine HCL test below, which is a supplement you can buy in the health-food shop. If you are already on medications, check with your doctor that they are compatible with betaine HCL.

BETAINE HCL TEST

🏠 *Home*

Take 1 capsule of betaine HCL before the last mouthful of your main meal (one that contains protein and fat, not mostly carbohydrate, such as salad, soup or fruit). Any burning sensation or indigestion means you have plenty of HCL already or, again, that you may have a stomach ulcer and should consult your doctor. So, to be clear, one way or another, if it burns, stop the test at this point.

If you don't have any burning sensation, however, then take two capsules of betaine HCL the next day, followed by three capsules the following day. If you still have no burning sensation, then you need more HCL and should keep adding a capsule to each meal until you get heartburn or some sign of irritation. When you reach this point, take one capsule less at your next meal.

If you are going to have a meal made up of mainly carbohydrate (no dairy or animal protein) then take half the dose. Any time you experience any irritation, reduce your dose by 1 capsule each meal until it no longer occurs. Your body will then have rebalanced its stomach acid levels.

Enzymes

We each have around 3,000 different varieties of enzymes, which are involved in vast numbers of metabolic processes and functions, including helping you to digest food, repair and renew, as well as keep your immune system strong.[4]

As we age our levels of digestive enzymes decrease, so a 70-year-old has half the number of a 20-year-old. Enzymes are found naturally in raw or fermented foods, but are destroyed by cooking. Much of what we eat is cooked or processed, so the majority of our food nowadays is almost entirely lacking in enzymes. Low or non-existent levels make you age faster and put on weight so enzymes are essential for looking and feeling young. Low enzyme levels are also linked to chronic diseases, such as obesity, heart disease and certain forms of cancer.

So how to replace them? Certain foods can boost your reserves, but you can also take supplements to increase your supply more rapidly.

Enzyme aids

These are the single most important health assistants that no one has ever heard of. All the cells in your body need loads of enzymes to keep them strong and healthy, and to keep up with their building and repair work, but after the age of about 25 the body stops producing them naturally, so you need to supplement to boost your immune system.

There are three basic types of enzyme aids:

1. Natural enzymes

Found in raw organic foods – especially fruits and vegetables but also unpasteurized milk, egg yolks, sauerkraut and kimchi. Natural enzymes are good for the immune system, joints and arteries.

2. Digestive enzymes

Found mainly in your gut, digestive enzymes help minimize indigestion, acid reflux, bloating and gas. There are three main digestive enzymes in the body:

- Amylase breaks down carbohydrates
- Lipase breaks down fats
- Protease breaks down proteins

All three enzymes are produced in the pancreas, and found naturally in raw fruits and vegetables, sprouted seeds, raw nuts, wholegrains and legumes. Most supplements will contain these three plus a combination of additional supporting enzymes, including:

- **Lactase:** Breaks down the lactose in milk and other dairy products (destroyed during pasteurization)
- **Maltase:** Breaks down sugars to form glucose
- **Sucrase:** Converts sugars into glucose and fructose
- **Pectinase:** Breaks down the cell walls of fruits to release more juice
- **Renin:** Helps digest proteins specifically found in milk

- **Cellulase:** Breaks down cellulose fibres (like celery), boosts digestion of proteins and controls blood sugar levels and cholesterol

3. Systemic enzymes

Systemic enzymes go after rogue proteins in your bloodstream and soft tissues. They mend and repair the body, remove toxins, clean the blood and liver, and reduce inflammation, as well as help with scarring, boost white blood cells, dissolve plaque in your arteries and control candida. Take systemic enzymes in between meals on an empty stomach and check the supplement labels for an optimal combination.

- **Bromelain:** Found as a single supplement and also in pineapple, this breaks down proteins, is good for arthritis and inflammation, serves as a substitute for pepsin (in case of pancreatic problems) and has anticancer properties

- **Papain:** Found as a single supplement and also in papaya, this breaks down animal proteins, is good for flatulence and indigestion, and dissolves dead tissue

- **Nattokinase:** Breaks down fibrin proteins that build up blood clots and plaque on the artery walls

- **Peptidase and protease:** Balances pH levels, improves circulation and boosts the liver by removing toxins

- **Seaprose-S:** Nature's antibiotic, this wipes out bacteria (including salmonella), reduces inflammation and breaks down mucus

- **Catalase:** One of the most effective antioxidant enzymes

- **Serrapeptase:** Reduces the viscosity of mucus, speeding up drainage. It is also good for joints and sinuses, and boosting general immunity

Action plan

→ **Take digestive enzymes with each meal:** Enzymes come in different combinations, so read the labels and pick what works for your specific issues.

→ **For ulcers:** Take DGL (deglycyrrhizinated liquorice)[5] in a chewable form, not as a capsule, because saliva makes it work more effectively.

→ **Portion control:** If you regularly overeat and feel overfull after meals then invest in a Full Stop Bowl (fullstopbowl. com), a stomach-sized and shaped bowl designed to encourage you to eat only what your stomach can actually hold – which is not a lot. Genius!

→ **Improve your eating habits:** Chew each mouthful at least 20 times before swallowing. Chewing produces saliva (which contains amylase) and starts the digestive process efficiently, enabling the food to be broken down thoroughly. Swallowing down large lumps of food too quickly causes problems for the gut, as undigested food ferments, creating toxins and gases that irritate the stomach lining; it also prevents absorption of nutrients and creates digestive problems.

Chapter 4

The Small Intestine: Your Food Blender

'A good eater must be a good man; for a good eater must have a good digestion, and a good digestion depends upon a good conscience.'

BENJAMIN DISRAELI

Your small intestine digests more of your food than the stomach and 70–90 per cent of your intestinal parasites live here. The small intestine is as wide as your thumb and approximately 5.5m (18ft) long, and is made up of three separate sections: the duodenum, the jejunum and the ileum. This is where the food that has already been broken down in your stomach is processed further, mixing with bile from the liver and juices from the pancreas. Around 95 per cent of the food you put in your mouth is digested here, with useful nutrients separated out from unusable waste products. Food stays in the small intestine for one to four hours, before moving on to the large intestine for further processing.

A healthy small intestine is all about controlling your bacteria levels, and mucus build-up on the walls can cause havoc and deplete your energy levels. If you have bloating, gas and loose bowel movements, and regularly fall asleep soon after eating, you may well have a small intestine issue such as candida, IBS (irritable bowel syndrome) or SIBO (small intestinal bacteria overgrowth). Bad breath is often an indicator you may have a problem.

SIBO BACTERIA TEST

🏠 *Home*

Gut bacteria excrete high levels of hydrogen and methane, which are then exhaled by your lungs and so can be measured. Available online (biohealthlab.com/patients), this simple breath test can tell you whether or not you have an overgrowth of bacteria.

SMALL INTESTINE BIOPSY

✚ *Doctor*

Your doctor may recommend this test. You swallow a small capsule attached to a long tube, which picks up a piece of tissue specimen and brings it back for sampling.

Bacteria

The bacteria in your gut weigh around 1kg (2lbs). You are never alone. In fact, there are 10 times more bacteria in your gut than there are cells in your body, and the balance of 'good' and 'bad' bacteria has a huge impact on how you feel and how your body functions. Gut bacteria are essential for an efficient food breakdown but, increasingly, research is proving that bacteria can also influence everything from depression and anxiety to immunity,[1] so you need the right ones working for you. Eating a poor diet and taking too many antibiotics can destroy the 'good' bacteria, allowing fungal infection to overwhelm your gut and multiply.

Candida is one of the most common, and trickiest, funguses to eliminate in the body, but rarely takes hold unless it is working hand-in-hand with an overgrowth of bacteria.[2] Candida spreads rapidly and develops root-like tendrils that can penetrate tissues and glands. It feeds on sugar and as sugar consumption has increased in recent decades, so has the growth of candida. The destruction of 'friendly' bacteria in the gut following repeated courses of antibiotics, the contraceptive pill, chlorinated tap water and a sugary diet all help 'bad' bacteria' to flourish exponentially and candida to multiply, so if you have candida, you have a bacteria problem, too.

CANDIDA TEST

 Home

Most of us have candida to some degree, although in many cases it doesn't cause a problem. Funguses can cause athlete's foot, thrush or ringworm, but there are other less obvious symptoms too, including exhaustion and gut and urinary tract infections (UTIs). This simple test is an effective way to check for candida.

1. Put out a fresh glass of water before going to bed.

2. First thing in the morning, briefly rinse your mouth, swallow, then gather some saliva and spit into the glass of water (be sure to spit out saliva, not mucus).

3. Keep an eye on the water for 30 minutes, paying particular attention in the first few minutes.

4. Refer to the illustration below and, if you have candida overgrowth, you will notice:

   - Strings (legs) hanging down from the saliva (1)

   - Cloudy specks suspended in the water (2)

   - Heavy-looking saliva at the bottom of the glass (3)

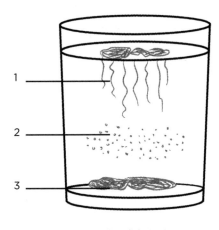

Candida test

TOP TIPS

- *Grapefruit seed extract wipes out candida and thrush. Take three to six drops in water daily after each meal.*

- *Allicin, a compound in garlic, is a powerful antibacterial agent and an effective remedy for candida and other fungal infections. Eat it raw on an empty stomach.*

HELICOBACTER PYLORI TEST

✚ *Doctor*

Helicobacter pylorus is a little-known bacterium found in the stomachs of more than two-thirds of the world's population. It is picked up from contaminated water or food, or from contact with the bodily fluids of infected people.

You may not have any symptoms, but *Helicobacter pylori* can be a major cause of sores, ulcers and even cancer in the lining of your stomach. It is the only bacteria able to survive in stomach acid, and side-effects include heartburn, bad breath, bloating and flatulence.

Your doctor can order a stool test to check if this is a problem for you and the usual cure for it is a prescription of antibiotics.

Microbiome

The gut isn't just where you process food, but is now considered a metabolic organ every bit as important as your heart or your liver. Research indicates that the immune system is heavily affected by the balance of good and bad bacteria in the gut.[3] 'Bad' bacteria cannot multiply and cause harm if they are kept in control by 'good' bacteria.

Scientific opinion is currently in its infancy, but it is clear that much of the state of our health is down to the trillions of microbes that live in the gut, breaking down food into nutrients and feeding themselves in the process.

In essence, the gut debate seems to be about the colonization of our world by microbes. They have set up shop in every crack and crevice of this planet we call home. They are invisible to the human eye but extremely hardy and can adapt to the toughest environments: darkness, heat, cold, damp, humidity and even no water at all.

Your gut is host to innumerable viruses, yeasts, bacteria, algae, moulds, funguses, archaea and protists (ever heard of the last two organisms? Me neither!), alongside hordes of other life forms you probably never knew existed. The vast majority of microbes live in your gut, colon and small intestine, but they are also all over your skin, and in your mouth, nose, stomach, lungs and vagina. Everywhere really. The only places they don't seem to colonize extensively are in the blood and lymph fluid.

Microbe minutiae

There are an estimated 100 trillion microbes living alongside and inside you. As a group, microbes are described as your 'microbiota' and the term 'microbiome' refers to your own personal microbe ecosystem – made up of individual varieties and quantities of microbe types specific to you.

What's in your gut is not thought to be a random muddle of microbes, but a particular set that have particular functions and purpose, even if medical researchers aren't currently quite clear about what they do or why.

Hundreds of thousands of different microbes have been identified and although only around 1,000 of them are found in humans, the same ones pop up time and time again. On average, each of us has a combination of around 160 bacteria types making up our microbiome[4] and each area of the body plays host to different microbes that have adapted to their particular environment. Skin microbes tend to be similar in all of us but very different, for example, from the microbes found in the gut.

So your individual microbiome is like a snowflake or fingerprint – similar but different – and once you've developed your own collection of microbes in early childhood, they don't change much.

The foundation of a healthy microbiome starts at birth and is built up over the following two years. You inherit around eight million microbiome genes from your parents, as well as picking them up from other people, topped up by additions from your environment and daily diet. The only things that can dramatically change your microbiome are losing or putting on weight, changing your diet, moving to a different country or wiping it out with antibiotics.

The key to wellbeing, to mental health, to youth and vitality and to most other happy things lies in the quality and diversity of the microbes in your gut garden. It's all about the terrain. An overload of processed foods, chemicals, pesticides and antibiotics creates a barren, rocky garden. If you want to get healthy, get gut gardening. Remove any rocks and dig out the weeds. Fertilize the soil with prebiotics and fibre; seed it with probiotics and your health will bloom.

Probiotics, probiotics, probiotics

Current research shows that if the balance of your gut microbiome is upset, health issues arise. Studies have shown that obesity, asthma, IBS, leaky gut, diabetes and some autoimmune diseases are likely to be linked to microbial disturbance.[5-6] The microbiome is thought to affect your mood, sleep patterns and anxiety levels, and some bacteria can throw your hormones out of balance.

Probiotics are the current buzzword for all things gut related, supplementing conventional medical treatment, though the jury is still out on whether they work or not. Some trials have shown that probiotics positively affect a wide range of health issues, such as anxiety and depression,[7] candida, allergies, IBS and Crohn's disease, and the hope is that they can be specifically developed to address and resolve particular health issues.

Other studies state that 99 per cent of the microbes that live in your gut are anaerobic, which means they are unable to use or eat oxygen. In addition, all the fermented foods and the bottles of probiotics we buy in the shops only contain bacteria that need oxygen to live. Overall, this means that probiotics are incompatible with the majority of your gut guests and can only affect around 1 per cent of your microbes positively.[8]

On top of this, in order to actively impact the gut microbiome, the bacteria in your probiotics need to be able to survive the strong gastric acid and bile in your stomach, and travel to the small and large intestine, where most of the gut bacteria colonies are located, and not get flushed straight through the GI tract.

Probiotics are expensive, so make sure you do your research and read the label carefully before buying. Higher numbers are better, so look for a count of 50 billion or more in each dose and as many different strains as possible – although a few strategically targeted strains can also work well. And if you're looking for a good all-round probiotic, choose *Lactobacillus* and *Bifidobacterium* plus additional strains according to the issue you want to deal with (see the table below). *Lactobacillus acidophilus* and *Lactobacillus plantarum* are the superstar strains.

Which probiotic?	
Health issue	**Strain**
Eczema	*Bifidobacterium bifidum, Bifidobacterium lactis, Lactococcus lactis, Escherichia coli*
Food allergies	*Escherichia coli, Lactobacillus paracasei*
Immunity	*Lactobacillus plantarum, Bacillus circulans*
After antibiotics	*Enterococcus mundtii, Lactobacillus plantarum, Lactobacillus brevis, Lactobacillus* strains, *Bifidobacterium* strains
Gastroenteritis	*Lactobacillus casei*
Intestinal hyper-permeability	*Lactobacillus plantarum*
Vaginal candidiasis (thrush)	*Lactobacillus rhamnosus, Lactobacillus reuteri, Lactobacillus fermentum*
Urinary tract infection, mastitis and throat infection	*Lactobacillus rhamnosus, Lactobacillus reuteri, Lactobacillus fermentum, Lactobacillus salivarius, Streptococcus salivarius*
Lactose intolerance	*Lactobacillus acidophilus*
After non-steroidal anti-inflammatory drug (NSAID)	*Escherichia coli* strain[9]
Intestinal microbial imbalance	*Lactobacillus johnsonii, Lactobacillus* strain, *Lactobacillus* GG[10]

Which probiotic? (continued)	
Health issue	**Strain**
Irritable bowel syndrome (IBS)	*Bifidobacterium infantis, Escherichia coli, Lactobacillus plantarum, Lactobacillus reuteri protectis, Bifidobacterium lactis, Lactobacillus rhamnosus, Lactobacillus acidophilus, Enterococcus faecium* *Bacillus coagulans, Saccharomyces cerevisiae*
Traveller's tummy/diarrhoea	*Lactobacillus rhamnosus, Lactobacillus plantarum*
Antibiotic-associated diarrhoea	*Lactobacillus reuteri protectis, LGG and Saccharomyces boulardii*
Radiation-induced diarrhoea	*Lactobacillus casei*
Crohn's disease	*Escherichia coli strain, Lactobacillus plantarum*
Protection against colon cancer	*Enterococcus faecium*, Lactic acid bacteria
Ulcerative colitis	*Lactobacillus acidophilus, Lactobacillus plantarum, Escherichia coli strain, Bifidobacterium*
Peptic ulcer disease	*Lactobacillus acidophilus*
Protection against atrophy	*Lactobacillus rhamnosus GG*
Hypercholesterolemia and cardiovascular diseases	*Enterococcus faecium, Lactobacillus plantarum, Propionibacterium freudenreichii, Lactobacillus plantarum*
Depression	*Lactobacillus helveticus, Bifidobacterium longum*
Anti-inflammatory	*Faecalibacterium prausnitzii*

Which probiotic?	
Health issue	**Strain**
Cholesterol	*Lactobacillus amylovorus, Bifidobacterium breve, Bifidobacterium lactis*
Weight loss	*Christensenella, Bifidobacterium breve, Lactobacillus rhamnosus, Lactobacillus gasseri*
Healthy gut	*Lactobacillus fermentum*
Stomach acid and after antibiotics	*Lactobacillus acidophilus, Bacillus coagulans, Saccharomyces boulardii, Lactobacillus rhamnosus* (proven to survive stomach acid)

It's worth noting that of the probiotics listed above, *Lactobacillus GG* is the most clinically studied, and *Lactobacillus acidophilus* and *Bifidobacterium longum* can both survive hot temperatures and don't need to be kept in the fridge.

What's the difference – probiotics and prebiotics?

Probiotics are live bacteria, and taking them can be a bit hit and miss as we don't really know which strain is missing in the gut; they are also easily destroyed and can pass out of the body very rapidly. Prebiotics, however, are a sort of plant fibre that feed the good bacteria and are effectively gut fertilizers. More bacteria mean better health – both physical and mental.

Action plan

→ **Take probiotics and supplement daily:** Check the packaging of any probiotics to make sure you are buying the right strains for your specific problem. Also check they are strains that will survive the journey through your stomach acid, and also be aware that some need to live in the fridge once opened.

→ **Use probiotics after antibiotics:** Taking antibiotics is like setting off a bomb inside your intestinal tract – it nukes the entire environment, allowing bad bacteria to multiply uncontrollably, so take large doses of probiotics immediately after finishing any course of antibiotics.[11]

→ **Take prebiotics:** This is the food that the healthy gut bacteria like for lunch! Keep the probiotics fed with prebiotics daily (you can buy them in small sachets) and their numbers will multiply along with your good bacteria.[12]

→ **Boost your digestive enzymes to break down mucus:** Digestive enzymes can help, particularly bromelain and papain (see Chapter 3, page 41).

→ **Visit a herbalist:** The herb mullein dissolves mucus efficiently, as does Greek mastic gum, but you'll need to visit a herbalist for correct dosing.

→ **Take comfrey:** This heals the gut membrane, improving digestion. Make a tea from 14g (1/2oz) fresh chopped leaves steeped in boiling water and then strained. Add a little fresh ginger, cinnamon or mint for optimal efficacy.

→ **Drink slippery elm tea:** This calms inflammation of the small intestine and relieves IBS.

→ **Drink plenty of water:** Water keeps your gut tubes lubricated and smooth.

→ **Boost your vitamins A and D:** Eat liver to protect the mucus membrane of the gut (see the Appendix).

➜ **Eat more antibacterial foods:** Garlic, honey and sauerkraut prevent the growth of candida, fungus and yeast infections, and can improve gut health. You might also like to try:

- Oregano oil (preferably the pure *Oreganum vulgare* from the mountains of Turkey and Lebanon) has been scientifically proven to stop candida in its tracks. Take three to four drops in water twice daily.[13]

- Aloe vera, turmeric and apple cider vinegar are all effective antimicrobial natural remedies.

- Ginger tea, made with a few slices of the fresh root steeped in hot water, is an effective remedy for viruses and bacteria.

- Raw organic honey contains live enzymes that release hydrogen peroxide, which kills germs and viruses.

BONE BROTH

🌿 *Remedy*

Bone broth (a clear soup of boiled-up organic beef or chicken bones cooked with water, garlic and onions for 24 hours in a slow cooker) can help to heal any damage to your intestines, as well as soothe IBS and leaky gut. Drink a cupful every night on an empty stomach before bed.

Overcoming other common gut issues

There are a number of gut problems that can upset your digestive system, but generally it is possible to resolve them with natural remedies combined with simple changes to your diet and lifestyle.

Leaky gut

Leaky gut is a condition whereby wear and tear on the lining of the intestine (as a consequence of repeated bouts of candida, parasites, overuse of antibiotics, gluten intolerance or the overgrowth of certain bacteria) make it overly permeable. Incompletely digested foods can then penetrate the gut wall and foods which wouldn't normally cause a problem trigger an allergic reaction. Toxins that would otherwise be contained in the bowel leak into the bloodstream and the lymphatic system causing inflammation and exhaustion. Other symptoms include fluid retention, weight gain, joint pain and bloating.

A combination of leaky gut, 'bad' bacteria build-up and low stomach acid may be behind any symptoms of IBS.

LEAKY GUT TEST

✚ *Doctor*

A doctor or naturopath can arrange for you to have a urine test to measure the ability of two sugar molecules, mannitol and lactulose, to pass through the lining of your small intestine. This will give you a clear picture of the permeability of your gut. If lactulose, which has the larger molecules, ends up in your urine, your gut is officially leaky.

Action plan

→ **Cut out:** Where possible avoid alcohol, Ibuprofen or any other non-prescription medications, as these can cause inflammation and damage the gut.

→ **Supplement:** Leaky gut creates mineral and vitamin deficiencies, so supplement daily with digestive enzymes (see Chapter 3, page 39), vitamin B6 and zinc. Digestive enzymes reduce food allergy and intolerance issues and help with production of HCL and digestion; vitamin B6 boosts stomach acid and zinc helps intolerance symptoms. You might also want to add L-Glutamine, and butyric acid (1,200mg daily) can help heal the gut, but dosage is important, so check with a nutritionist to ensure the supplements are tailored to you.

→ **Go gluten-free:** Cut out gluten entirely for a week and keep a food diary to check if your symptoms improve. More and more people are developing sensitivity to wheat, rye, barley and other grains. These grains contain gluten and gliadins, which are hard to digest and can allow undigested foods and toxins to slip through, causing inflammation and a raised immune response.

→ **Check for candida or bacterial infections:** Cut out all sugar and dairy from your diet. Keep a food diary so you can track any changes.

→ **Take probiotics:** Probiotics help digest your food, deal with any 'bad' bacteria in your gut and boost your immune system.

→ **Soothe your gut walls:** Aloe vera juice, turmeric and ginger all have beneficial soothing qualities.

➜ **Make some bone broth:** Full of collagen, proline and glycine that work together to heal gut issues (see page 55).

Your ileocaecal valve (ICV)

Connecting the small and the large intestines, the ileocecal valve should open and close quickly, as digested food moves out from the small intestine and into the large intestine. The ICV operates like a one-way street and prevents food accidentally washing back into the small intestine. However, dehydration, emotional stress, fizzy drinks, overeating and not chewing your food sufficiently can all cause it to get stuck and result in lower back pain, constipation, right shoulder pain and headaches.

ICV REMEDY

🌿 *Remedy*

If you have tried and failed to relieve your symptoms, it is worth attempting the following simple home remedy to reset the ICV:

1. Put your right hand on the bone of your right hip, keeping your little finger on its inside edge. Your hand will now be over the ileocecal valve.

2. Put your left hand in the same place on your left hip, inside the bone. (Your left hand will now be over the Houston valve; if this valve isn't working properly, you may have a continual urge to defecate and it can be reset at the same time as the ICV.)

3. Press your fingers in firmly and move the fingers of both hands upwards, towards your ribcage, while taking deep breaths.

4. Shake your fingers when you reach that point.

5. Breathe out, lift your fingers and go back to where you started. Repeat the movement four more times.

6. End the treatment by dragging your fingers downwards, whilst pressing firmly.

Reduce your allergy load

Over 20 per cent of us are affected by mild food reactions or intolerances,[14] and milk, wheat or gluten, sugar, seafood, alcohol, coffee, nuts, soya and eggs often play a part in triggering gut problems.

If you have digestive issues, you might need to try an elimination diet to work out where the problem lies. Immunoglobulin E (IgE) antibodies in your blood indicate life-threatening allergies (e.g. peanuts or wasp stings), and come with severe and immediate reactions – swelling, breathing difficulties, anaphylactic shock. Immunoglobulin G (IgG) antibody testing is for food sensitivities, some of which you may not even be aware you suffer from yet have adverse effects on you. Once identified, you can begin to address any problems.

FOOD ALLERGY TEST

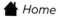 *Home*

Reactions to foods will usually show up as a change in your pulse rate and you'll be recording your bpm (beats per minute) in this test (see Chapter 1, page 23).

1. First thing in the morning, before you eat or drink, take your pulse, holding and counting for a full minute. Make sure you are relaxed when you take it. Write down your bpm.

2. Chew the food that you want to test for at least 30 seconds, but don't swallow it.

3. With the food still in your mouth, take your pulse again for a further minute and record your bpm.

4. Spit out the food and rinse your mouth with water.

5. A rise of 6bpm or more indicates a stress reaction in your body, so avoid that food for at least a month before testing again.

6. After a month, gradually reintroduce small amounts of the food to see if you're able to tolerate it in lesser quantities.

Don't test a second food until your pulse has returned to its early morning baseline.

TOP TIP

If you are testing eggs, make sure that you test your reaction to the yolk and white separately, as the whites more often trigger a reaction than the yolk.

Action plan

→ **Get allergy tested:** If, after seeing your doctor, you're unable to pinpoint the issue, then consider food allergy testing with a qualified nutritionist.

→ **Book in for NAET (Nambudripad's Allergy Elimination Technique) or health kinesiology:** Both therapies can help to identify and desensitize allergic reactions.

Parasites

We all have parasites living in our gut, but the growth of the wrong type can mean that you don't get the full benefit of the food that you eat. Most parasites are caught from undercooked meats, unwashed vegetables and fruits, and contaminated water and foods. There are thousands of different types of parasites and the only way to test for them reliably is via your doctor or nutritionist, but some of the indicators of a parasite problem include:

- Constipation, diarrhoea, gas, a bloated stomach or other symptoms of IBS
- Your digestion not being the same since a bout of food poisoning
- Trouble falling asleep or waking frequently during the night
- Eczema, skin irritations or unexplained skin rashes
- Continually biting your nails to the quick
- Grinding your teeth in your sleep
- Pain or aching in your muscles or joints
- Often tired, exhausted, depressed or generally apathetic
- Not feeling satisfied or full after eating
- Iron-deficiency anaemia

CHECKING FOR PARASITES

✚ *Doctor*

> A live blood analysis test via a naturopath or nutritionist, or a stool test with your doctor, will show whether or not you have parasites in your system.

Action plan

→ **Wash your hands more:** Minimize your possibility of catching parasites by washing your hands frequently, particularly after going to the bathroom and always after patting animals or gardening.

→ **Avoid sushi and pork products:** If you're trying to get rid of parasites, cut down on raw fish, as it often contains infected larvae if not prepared properly. Undercooked pork has also been flagged as a source of parasites since biblical times, and even freezing doesn't destroy the worms.

→ **Natural parasite cleansing supplements:** Hippocrates Health Institute's FCR (Freedom Cleanse Restore), a course of herb-filled capsules, is an excellent remedy. Once you've finished the course, take a two-week break and then do another course to ensure any unhatched parasites are also destroyed. Health stores offer a range of similar products.

→ **Zap parasites:** For a lifetime's management of potential parasite problems try Dr Hulda Clark's Zapper. Dr Clark researched the links between parasites and disease, and developed a small black box that pulses specific frequencies through the body to destroy parasites and pathogens, but leaves healthy cells unaffected.[15-16]

➔ **Ayurveda herbs:** *Mimosa pudica* powder is brilliant for wiping out parasites if taken for three months. Take ½ teaspoon twice a day, twice a week initially, and slowly increase the dosage to one teaspoon a day.

➔ **Increase your daily use of antiparasitic foods and spices:** Eat more garlic, thyme, chilli, turmeric and ginger. Coconut oil is also antifungal.

➔ **Create balance:** Up the levels of HCL in your stomach (see Chapter 3, page 37) and follow up with probiotics.

TOP TIP

Giardia is a particularly disruptive parasite and can trigger debilitating health problems. It is hard to shift, but herbalist Susan Koten has developed a spray that is effective in eradicating the issue (willowherbalcentre.co.uk).

Chapter 5

The Large Intestine:
Your Food Compactor

*'Happiness for me is largely
a matter of digestion.'*

LIN YUTANG

The large intestine is a 1.5m (5ft) long, U-shaped, ropey tube, running from the bottom right side of your torso up to your ribs, across to the left side of your body and down again to the bottom left side, across to the middle and finishes by connecting to your rectum. Here the food – which probably hit your mouth 24 hours earlier – finally leaves your body. The large intestine's job is to wring all the remaining water and nutrients out of any food that comes its way and turn it all into compact faeces or stools. In your lifetime, it will process approximately 50 tons of food.

When things start going wrong, inflammation is usually the result and this can lead to a range of symptoms – including stomach pain, cramps, bloating, flatulence and frequent diarrhoea or constipation. This could point to any one of the many colon-linked diseases from IBS to Crohn's disease, ulcerative colitis or colorectal cancer. For this reason, it is vital that any changes in your bowel movements or stools are reported to your doctor.

COLON HEALTH CHECK-UP

✚ *Doctor*

Your doctor is likely to request a stool sample, physically examine your stomach for enlarged organs, order blood tests and may refer you to a specialist for a colonoscopy (which looks thoroughly at your colon walls and can take a biopsy for testing).

Action plan

→ **Eat less red meat and avoid any cured or smoked meats:** These foods are known to increase risk of colorectal cancer.[1] Eat more fruit and vegetables for plant antioxidants and fibre.

→ **Up your selenium levels:** High levels of selenium are linked to low colon cancer risks, so increase your intake of Brazil nuts, salmon, onions, oats and brown rice.[2] Olive, flaxseed and avocado oil are also beneficial, as is L-Glutamine and raw pumpkin seeds.[3]

→ **Book in for a colonic:** Colonics flush out any build-up of mucus, plaque and toxins, and provide an instant cleanse for your large intestine. Afterwards, you're likely to notice feeling more energized and have clearer skin. Follow up with a daily probiotic to repopulate your colon with good bacteria.

→ **If colonics aren't for you:** A natural herbal colon-cleansing supplement can help break down the mucus on the colon wall, remove toxins and clean out old waste. Ask a nutritionist or naturopathic doctor for their recommendations.

ENEMA CLEANSE

🌿 *Remedy*

An enema is a way of keeping the lower part of your colon clean and healthy by flushing it out with purified water. You regularly wash the outside of your body, but cleaning the inside is just as important. Enemas hydrate your colon, at the same time as getting rid of infections, bacteria and toxins.

Enemas are inexpensive and easy to do at home in the bathroom. All you need is an enema bag, one teaspoon of coconut oil and 2 litres (approx. 4 pints) of distilled water.

1. Open up the enema bag and move the clip on the tube leading from the bag to the closed position so that it pinches the tube shut.

2. Fill the bag with room temperature distilled water.

3. Hold the bag over the sink and open the clip until the water flows out and there is no air in the tube.

4. Close the clip again and then hang the bag at door-handle height. If you hang the bag any higher the water may flow too fast, any lower and it may not flow at all. Like the three bears, you need to get the height 'just right'.

5. Lubricate the last 5cm (2in) of the tube with coconut or olive oil (make sure it's not a petroleum-based product or anything not designed for internal use) and then lie down on a towel on the floor on your left side. Keep your left leg straight and lift your right leg, bent at the knee, towards your chest.

6. Take a few deep breaths and focus on relaxing your body before gently inserting the first 5cm (2in) of the tube into your rectum.

7. Push the clip on the tube to the 'open' position and feel the water flowing into you. Try to hold as much water as you can, hopefully leaving just 1.5cm (½in) of water in the bag at the end. Then close the clip again and remove the tube.

8. Hold onto the water for several minutes (although the first few times this may only be a matter of seconds) to allow the water to hydrate your colon and loosen any waste.

9. Roll onto your back and bend both of your knees towards your chest, gently massaging your stomach for two minutes. Then do the same thing on your right side and a further two minutes on your left side.

10. When you need to let the water go, sit on the toilet for a few minutes. It will all come flooding out!

11. After an initial water enema, add 110g (3¾ oz) of fresh wheatgrass or aloe vera juice with 85g (3oz) of blue-green algae to the last 2–3cm (¾ –1¼in) of water. This is a direct way of getting nutrition into your colon walls and the longer you can hold it in the better.

12. When you've finished, rinse the bag and tube in hot water. Hang it up to dry and replace every few months.

13. Make sure you that you take a capsule of probiotics afterwards to stimulate the growth of the good bacteria in your colon (see Chapter 4, page 49).

14. For a thorough clean, do an enema daily for a week and then repeat twice a month.

More on gut bacteria

We explored the benefits of good bacteria in the previous chapter, but they also play a vital role in the health of your large intestine.

When you're a baby, the majority of your bacteria are *Bifidobacterium*, which coat the gut preventing the attachment of any pathogens. As adults, most of our gut inhabitants are bacteria (rather than fungi, yeast or viruses), and a balance of *Bacteroidetes* and *Firmicutes* usually make up the majority of these bacteria and regulate how much fat you absorb and where you store it.

STOOL THERAPY

Research into overweight mice has shown that they have considerably higher levels of Firmicutes *and lower levels of* Bacteroidetes.[4] *Skinny mice have the opposite results. When researchers transferred faeces from overweight mice into the intestinal tracts of skinny mice, they found that their bacteria ratios overrode the natural tendency of the skinny mice, so that they became overweight as a result.*

Research into stool therapy (using human faecal implants to heal serious gut issues) also met with success and faecal pills are available over the Internet,[5] but it's worth noting that these studies' participants also inherited mental and obesity issues from their donors, so do be cautious about your supplier.

Gut diversity reduces after the age of 65, probably because the immune system weakens, but also because of changes in eating habits, overuse of medical prescriptions and digestive tract issues, including constipation. In addition, *Bifidobacterium* levels naturally decline and *Proteobacterium* levels increase, suggesting that supplementation could be essential.

Action plan

→ **Minimize your stress levels:** From a microbe's point of view, stress upsets your digestion and reduces your *Bacteroidetes*, which increases your risk of weight gain and makes you more stressed – and on it goes.

→ **Eat more vegetables:** Bacteroidetes love fruits, beans and pulses, so eat lots of them, Firmicutes thrive on fat and sugar, so eat less if you want to avoid weight gain.

→ **Eat widely:** Diversity of food equals diversity of gut bacteria.

→ **Map your gut:** Mapmygut.com is a US study that will analyse the microbe content of your faeces for a small fee.

TOP TIP

If you want fewer Firmicutes *and more* Bacteroidetes *bacteria then feed your good bacteria with the full-spectrum prebiotic Prebiotin™, which works throughout the large intestine.*

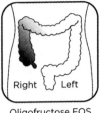 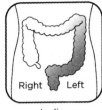 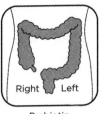

Right Left	Right Left	Right Left
Oligofructose FOS	Inulin	Prebiotin

*Prebiotics in the large colon: the darker areas
indicate where each type works*

BOWEL TEST

 Home

Assessing your faeces and your regularity (what your stools look like and how often you go to the lavatory) might not be polite conversation at the dinner table, but becoming more aware of your bowel movements will provide you with an at-a-glance indicator of your lifestyle and the state of your gut health.

Bowel health checklist:

- There should be no discomfort or straining when you go to the loo and no smell of gas.

- Stools should come out easily, smoothly and all in one piece.

- Stools should be 10–15cm (4–5½in) long and medium brown in colour. They shouldn't be smelly, stick to the lavatory bowl or float.

- If your poo floats, this could be due to too much fat or gas in your diet – usually from excess sugar, fizzy drinks or beans. It can also be a sign of poor absorption, lactose intolerance or coeliac disease – particularly if your stools look greasy and smell bad – in which case you need to book a check-up with your doctor.

- A very smelly stool can also be a sign of undigested food or waste that has been sitting in your bowel for a long time.

- Going to the loo two to three times a day is optimal, but anything from two to three times per day to two to three times per week is normal. Any changes to your normal pattern should be reported to your doctor.

Colour Analysis

Here's a guide to what your stools say about you:[6]

Very pale: Bile gives the stool its colour and lack of bile could be due to gallstones, liver problems or parasites; it can also indicate lactose intolerance.

Very dark: The stool has been sitting for some time in your intestine. Eating more fibre (from vegetables, fruit and wholegrains) and drinking more water should help the situation.

Greenish: Another sign that there is a lack of bile, where green foodstuffs are not being broken down and absorbed properly.

Yellowish: A sign of excess fat, which may indicate an absorption problem or possibly coeliac disease.

Red/purple: If there is fresh blood, this can be due to bleeding in the rectum, often from haemorrhoids. If the blood is darker and older in appearance, this can be a sign of bleeding in the upper digestive tract. If blood in the stool continues for more than a couple of days, or becomes regular, you should consult a doctor immediately.

Action plan

→ **Drink more water, eat more fibre:** Increasing the amount of water you drink and upping your fibre (e.g. well-cooked brown rice, oatmeal, prunes, kiwi fruit or flaxseeds) should produce at least one bowel movement a day and will avoid undigested waste sitting around in your gut.[7]

→ **Exercise:** A sedentary lifestyle can slow down your bowels so bring more movement into your day. (See also Chapter 20.)

→ **Sit properly:** Invest in a low stool to put your feet on when you use the lavatory. Bend slightly forwards from the waist to allow a smoother passage for elimination.

→ **Retrain your bowels**: A series of colonics with a professional colon therapist is the simplest way to clear backed-up faeces and get things moving again. If long-term constipation is a problem, investing in a clysmatic machine (bowel irrigation system) is a simple way to retrain your bowels to evacuate efficiently once more.

→ **Take slippery elm capsules:** This is a natural way to ease constipation.

Chapter 6

The Pancreas:
Your Blood Sugar Control

'Today, the world is so awash in sugar – it is such a staple of the modern diet, associated with all that is cheap and unhealthy.'

TOM REISS

This little-talked about organ sits behind the stomach and produces several important hormones – including insulin, glucagon, somatostatin and pancreatic polypeptide – all of which circulate in the blood. The pancreas also secretes pancreatic juices to neutralize acidity from the stomach, as well as sending digestive enzymes into the small intestine to further break down carbohydrates, proteins and lipids.

If your pancreas stops working properly and doesn't produce enough insulin, diabetes is ultimately the result. Your pancreas is meant to produce insulin and release it into your bloodstream, adjusting the amounts of glucose your body needs to work properly. So, although a raised blood sugar level is a sign of diabetes, the underlying cause is usually a leptin and insulin-signalling issue.

Leptin is produced in your fat cells and regulates appetite and weight gain by telling your brain when to start and stop eating (see Chapter 19, page 186). Leptin is responsible for the accuracy of your insulin-signalling pathway and if those signals fail, insulin resistance can lead to Type 2 diabetes.

Unlike Type 2 diabetes, Type 1 diabetes tends to affect young people and at present there is no known cure, though stem cell science is rapidly developing and has shown success in the field. Type 1 diabetes develops when the immune system, possibly triggered by an infection or virus, destroys the insulin-producing cells in the pancreas.

The good news is that if you catch the disease in the prediabetic stage, you can prevent it from developing by upping your exercise levels and changing your diet. Warning signs include weight gain, high blood pressure readings, low 'good' cholesterol and high triglycerides. If you're over 40 and a close relative also has diabetes, it's worth asking your doctor for a test.

PANCREATIC HEALTH

✚ *Doctor*

Blood tests, an X-ray or a CT scan will give your doctor a clear picture of your pancreas' health. High levels of amylase and lipase indicate pancreatitis, a severe inflammation of the pancreas in which white blood cell numbers rise dramatically.

A1C TESTING

✚ *Doctor*

Haemoglobin A1C testing by your doctor can identify your likelihood of developing Type 2 diabetes and alert you if you're prediabetic. It measures your blood sugars over two to three months. Elevated numbers indicates your sugars are poorly controlled and that you are becoming insulin resistant. Your A1C should be below 5.7 per cent. The higher your percentage, the greater your insulin resistance.

STOOL CHECK-UP

🏠 *Home*

If your stools float and are pale in colour, then you may have an absorption problem due to the pancreas not producing enough enzymes to break down the fats in your food. If you also have a stabbing pain in the stomach or feel sick straight after eating fatty foods, book an appointment for a check-up with your doctor.

Sugar – a major problem for your pancreas

When you load up on sugar, the pancreas struggles to produce enough insulin to process it and, over a long period of time, can stop working. Apart from being an addiction up there with smoking, alcohol and drugs, sugar is also linked to obesity – one of the main risk factors for diabetes.

Most fruits and vegetables contain natural sugar, but refined white or brown sugar is usually made from sugar cane or sugar beet – and much of it is genetically modified so best avoided.

TOP TIPS

- *Stevia is a small green leaf that is 200 times sweeter than sugar, so use it sparingly. It has been found to balance your blood sugar levels and boost metabolism, so can help with weight loss. Make sure you buy the crushed-up green powder rather than the highly processed white stevia.*

- *Change4Life's Food Scanner is an easy-to-use app that lets you scan your favourite supermarket buys and will give you the sugar content of each item, alongside what your consumption should be, based on your age.*

- *Keep a sugar diary and start to notice how much you're eating, then start to reduce the amount by cutting out what you can.*

Action plan

→ **Exercise:** This is one of the quickest ways to lower your insulin and leptin resistance. (See also Chapter 19.)

→ **Diet and weight management are key:** Create a healthier lifestyle by changing your eating habits to:

- Avoid sugar, particularly high fructose corn syrup, because fructose is thought to be behind the spiralling levels of insulin resistance, weight gain and Type 2 diabetes. Aim for a diet rich in fruits, vegetables, wholegrains, poultry, fish, seeds and nuts.

- Limit your alcohol intake as it is a sugar and can overload the pancreas.

- Take a daily probiotic (see Chapter 4, page 49).

- Avoid trans-fats found in fried foods, pies, margarine and ice cream, as they increase inflammation and can interfere with your insulin receptors.

- Cut out processed meats, as studies show that they can increase your risk of Type 2 diabetes by 19 per cent.[1]

- Eat more raw foods, as a low-calorie, enzyme-rich, raw-food diet has been shown to reverse Type 2 diabetes and renew the pancreas after four to six weeks.[2-3]

- Add digestive enzymes to help break down food effectively (see Chapter 3, page 39). Drinking two tablespoons of apple cider vinegar in a glass of warm water 15 minutes before eating will help boost enzyme production.

➔ **Consult a medical herbalist for a herbal tonic:**

- Goldenseal heals the pancreas by stimulating beta cells and lowering blood sugar levels.

- Liquorice root calms inflammation, and reduces swelling and pain.

TOP TIP

Pancreas Tonic is a scientifically trialled Ayurveda herbal supplement that positively affects glucose levels in Type 2 diabetes. Taking two capsules three times a day for three months significantly improved glucose control by 10–12 per cent.[4]

Chapter 7

The Liver:
Your Detox Factory

'Our bodies – including our brains – are not designed to function well on toxic foreign substances.'

JOAN LARSON

The liver is located on the right-hand side of your body, just below and behind your ribcage. It is the second largest organ in your body (after the skin) at an average weight of 1.6kg (3½lbs). Think of it as your toxin cleaning factory – removing harmful stuff and filtering your blood. The liver also helps keep your weight in check and when it's clean and happy, it speeds up your metabolism, helping to burn fat faster.

When your liver is struggling, it doesn't work as effectively. Your metabolism slows down and your body creates too much fat, building up the levels stored in the liver. When it contains more than 10 per cent fat, then you officially have a fatty liver. As a result, cholesterol levels rise, the body stops converting vitamin D properly and symptoms of PMS, acne, hair loss or female facial hair can develop. Blood sugar levels rise too, ultimately increasing your risk of Type 2 diabetes or other liver disease.

Alcoholism and heavy drinking is the number-one cause of a fatty liver, but a high-fat, high-sugar diet can also contribute to it, as can:

- Smoking

- Obesity

- Diabetes

- Hyperlipidaemia (high levels of fats in the blood)

- Genetic inheritance

- Rapid weight loss

- Certain medications, including aspirin, steroids, tamoxifen (Nolvadex) and tetracycline (Panmycin)

There are two types of fatty liver disease: alcohol-related liver disease (ARLD) and non-alcoholic fatty liver disease (NAFLD). You're at risk of the latter if you are overweight or obese, or have:

- High blood pressure

- High cholesterol

- Are over the age of 50

- Smoke

However, NAFLD is sometimes diagnosed in people without any of the above risk factors, including young children, and is more difficult to detect than ARLD until its latter stages. The good news is that there are many simple steps you can take to repair any damage and protect your liver from disease going forwards.

LIVER CHECK-UP

✚ *Doctor*

Your doctor can give you a good idea of how well your liver is functioning by doing a blood test. There are also inexpensive urine tests you can buy on the Internet.

Understanding liver test markers

To understand what your results mean, you need to know what liver test markers your doctor is looking for:

Albumin: Made in the liver, this protein carries vitamins, hormones and nutrients around the body, and keeps fluid from leaking out of the blood vessels. Albumin levels in the blood lower when the liver is damaged, or if your body is seriously shocked or severely inflamed; levels rise when you are dehydrated.

Globulin: Albumin makes up a bit more than half of the blood's protein and globulin, also produced in the liver, most of the rest. High levels indicate chronic inflammation or autoimmune disease. Low levels are a sign that your liver or kidneys are struggling.

Total protein: Proteins in your blood help the cells and tissues to grow and stay healthy. The total protein test measures your overall protein levels, including the combined amount of albumin and globulin, and can indicate a problem with your liver or kidneys.

Total bilirubin: This is an orange-yellow pigment that is created by excessive red blood cell destruction and can be measured to see how well your liver is functioning. High levels can cause jaundice; low levels may be associated with angina.

ALP: (Alkaline phosphatase): This enzyme is found mostly in the cells of the bones and liver, and can be used to help detect liver disease or bone disorders. If your levels are low, you may also be suffering from a lack of zinc; other symptoms include white spots on your nails, acne, a reduced sense of smell or taste, and being particularly prone to colds and flu.

AST (Aspartate aminotransferase): This enzyme is found in the heart, liver and skeletal muscles. When the heart, liver or muscle cells are injured, they release AST into the bloodstream.

ALT (Alanine aminotransferase): This enzyme is found mostly in the liver but also in smaller amounts in the kidneys, heart and muscles. When the liver is damaged, ALT is released into the bloodstream and readings increase.

GGT (Gamma-glutamyl transferase): This is another liver enzyme and when your liver is damaged, or bile flow is blocked, the concentration of GGT rises in the blood, indicating bile duct problems. It can also be a sign of drinking too much alcohol.

Action plan

→ **Boost your potassium levels:** Add more sweet potatoes, spinach and bananas to your diet, or supplement with around 4,700mg daily. Potassium lowers blood pressure and cholesterol levels at the same time as strengthening and cleaning your liver.

→ **Take a coffee enema:** The hepatic portal vein just inside your rectum goes directly to the liver. Doing a coffee enema will stimulate the liver to release bile, speeding up detoxification.

→ **Sweat it out:** A far-infrared sauna is the fastest and most effective way to get rid of toxins in your body, lightening the liver's load in the process. For home use, try a Firzone infrared blanket or dome sauna; these are relatively inexpensive and work well (firzone.co.uk).

→ **Support and strengthen:** If your liver is damaged, it will struggle to process the following foods:

- Meat and dairy (get your protein from beans and nuts as much as possible)

- Alcohol

- Processed carbohydrates (white bread, pasta, cakes, biscuits, crisps, sweets, ice cream, etc.)

- Salt

→ **Eat more raw foods and get juicing**: Beetroot, dark green leafy vegetables, onions, garlic, broccoli, cabbage and cauliflower all strengthen the liver. Drink juices made with beetroot, carrots, celery and lemon to support bile secretion and to help digest fats.

→ **Black seed oil:** This has been shown to reduce liver stress markers and improve recovery caused by chemical damage in processed foods.[1-2]

→ **Visit a herbalist for a liver cleansing, repairing and boosting tonic:** The most effective herbs include:

- Borututu bark

- Milk thistle

- Chanca piedra

- Celandine

- Chicory root

- Dandelion root

- Turmeric

- Peppermint

- Yellow dock root

➜ **Go to bed earlier:** Get seven to eight hours' sleep each night because the liver repairs itself at night between 1 and 3 a.m. (See also Chapter 22.)

➜ **Take steps to reduce your stress levels:** Research indicates that stress and fatigue can increase levels of the liver enzyme aspartate transaminase.[2]

➜ **Consult a nutritionist for an optimal nutrient package:** Typical liver-boosting supplements include folic acid, vitamins B3, B6, C and E, as well as glycine and taurine, alongside calcium.

➜ **Invest in an air purifier:** Whether you live in the city, where air pollution is rife, or the countryside, which is often full of pesticides sprayed on the fields, your liver struggles to deal with chemicals and pollution. Reduce the toxic load on your liver by choosing your household products carefully and maximizing the quality of the air that you breathe. (See also Chapter 24.)

CASTOR OIL PACKING

🌿 *Remedy*

Castor oil packing is a simple, traditional remedy that is believed to help detox the liver, as well as clear the skin and other digestive issues.

1. Start by covering your sofa or bed with an old towel to avoid staining.

2. Take a flannel, or similar-size piece of cloth, and soak it in castor oil.

3. Place the cloth on your skin in the area of the liver (right-hand side of your stomach under the ribs).

4. Place a piece of plastic wrap or plastic sheet over the top and cover with a hot-water bottle.

5. Lie back and relax for 30 minutes or more.

LIVER AND GALLBLADDER FLUSH

🌿 *Remedy*

An apple juice and lemon and olive oil gallbladder and liver cleanse is an inexpensive and effective way to clean your liver and gallbladder. The flush is simple to do and you can find the instructions on how to do it here: daradietz.org/Liver-Cleanse-Andreas-Moritz.pdf

Note: If you have gallstones, this is flush is probably not for you, particularly if you have symptoms such as pain in your abdomen, vomiting, nausea or blood in your stools.

The process works best as a preventative detox. Certain pharmaceutical drugs can interact with the grapefruit juice, causing low blood pressure and the possibility of fainting. Other side-effects can include dehydration and electrolyte imbalance, which may affect you if you have heart arrhythmia issues. Always consult your doctor before going ahead with the gallbladder and liver flush.

Chapter 8

The Gallbladder:
Your Bile Producer

'Growth in wisdom can be measured
precisely by decline in bile.'

FRIEDRICH NIETZSCHE

The gallbladder sits below the liver to the right and looks like a small deflated balloon. Its main tasks are to store excess bile (on average 480g/1lb) from the liver, and to absorb fat-soluble vitamins and nutrients. Dine out on heavy, greasy foods, pile on the pounds and it will struggle to function. If your cholesterol level rises, it can also trigger the formation of tiny stones that block the bile ducts.

Gallbladder health is all about increasing bile flow to make sure you are digesting fatty foods efficiently and absorbing fat-based nutrients. If you've had your gallbladder removed, then it's even more important to take steps to help yourself.

CHECK-UP

✚ *Doctor*

If you have any of the typical signs of gallbladder problems – pain in the right shoulder or your stomach, feeling sick, pain under your right ribs and pain that gets worse when you cough – then get checked by your doctor immediately. You will probably be offered an initial scan and often surgery.

Action plan

→ **Stimulate the gallbladder:** Acupuncture or acupressure can stimulate specific points with needles or pressure points to unblock, rebalance and re-energize the body. The liver and the gallbladder are paired in Traditional Chinese Medicine (TCM), so what you do to strengthen one, works on the other (see Chapter 18, page 147).

→ **Eat a gallbladder-friendly diet:** Avoid saturated fats and add in more fresh fruit and vegetables, wholegrains, lean meats, fish and low-fat dairy products.

→ **Eat more raw foods:** Raw foods boost your natural enzymes and help the digestive process.

→ **Supplement with gallbladder-strengthening enzymes and nutrients:**[1-3]

   ~ Lipase helps with fat digestion.

   ~ Ox bile helps digestion, as well as increases the levels of good bacteria and helps to break down fats.

- Beetroot juice and beet extract supplements, from the top of the beetroot plant, improve bile flow. Add in bile salts for extra punch.

- Artichokes contain caffeoylquinic acid, which promotes bile flow.

- Sauerkraut helps promote bile flow.

TOP TIP

If you've had your gallbladder removed, you will need to make up for the loss of bile by using bile salts to help your digestion and absorption of fats and fat-soluble vitamins.

Chapter 9

The Kidneys:
Your Hydration Control

*'But I know all about love already. I know
precious little about kidneys.'*

ALDOUS HUXLEY

Your kidneys are located at waist level towards your back; you
have two of them, but your body can still work effectively
with just one. The kidneys are the same shape as a kidney bean,
but 10–12cm (4–5in) long or the size of a small mobile phone.
Their job is to clean your blood, filtering 227 litres (60 gallons) a
day – nearly 9 litres (2½ gallons) an hour – and removing waste
into your urine, where it is then excreted from your body. The
kidneys also control your fluid and electrolyte levels and your
blood pressure, as well as making vitamin D and red blood cells.

Dehydration is a major issue for the health of your kidneys.
If you don't drink enough water each day, they stop working
properly, ultimately resulting in kidney stones and, more
seriously, prerenal failure. Prerenal failure is when the kidneys
don't receive enough blood to filter and can happen when
plaque narrows the blood vessels, or be triggered by sepsis,

heart attack or liver failure. The unhealthy fad for taking water pills to lose weight is also a contributor to more serious kidney problems.

QUICK KIDNEY TEST

 Home

Take a urine sample in the middle of the day (use a clean glass jar or specimen bottle). Your urine should be a clear pale yellow. If it's dark yellow, brown or pinkish, it indicates possible dehydration, infection or a more serious kidney issue. Your sample should smell very faintly of urine. Anything more pungent may also be a sign of kidney problems. Any blood in your urine may indicate an infection or kidney stones and should be checked by your doctor.

BLOOD AND URINE TESTS

✚ *Doctor*

High blood pressure readings can indicate a weakness in the kidneys, but urine tests are also accurate. One of the first signs that something is wrong is when there is a change in the amount and frequency of times you go to the bathroom. Your urine may get darker, you may feel cold all the time, you may find blood in your urine, or have a severe pain in your back or sides. Consult your doctor immediately if you have any of these symptoms as they can indicate infection.

Blood tests are the most comprehensive way of checking what's going on with your kidneys and can be carried out by your doctor.

Understanding your results

Urea: This indicates how well your kidneys are working. Urea is a waste product released by the liver that is filtered by the kidneys before being excreted from the body in your urine. If your kidneys are working well, they remove more than 90 per cent of the urea, so if you have high levels in your blood, there may be a problem.

Urea levels increase with age and high-protein diets can also raise your levels. Very low urea levels suggest that your liver is not processing urea effectively or that you are eating too little protein.

Creatinine: Found in the blood, this chemical is excreted by the kidneys via urine and is a marker of the excretion capability of the kidneys. The amount produced also depends on your gender, size, age and muscle mass, so creatinine concentrations will be slightly higher in men than in women and children.

eGFR (estimated Glomerular Filtration Rate): This measures the function of your kidneys by looking at the amount of blood that is filtered per minute. Glomeruli are tiny filters in your kidneys that allow waste products to be removed from the blood, while preventing the loss of important proteins and blood cells. When your kidneys are damaged or diseased, their filtration rate decreases and waste products begin to accumulate in the blood.

Glucose: A slight increase in blood glucose levels is a possible sign of prediabetes. Symptoms include excess hunger, thirst, frequent urination and visual changes. A high level of glucose can also indicate a deficiency of vitamin B1; a combination of high levels of cholesterol, triglycerides and glucose indicates a fatty liver problem.

Calcium: Although 99 per cent of calcium is in the bones, the rest is found in the blood, and these levels are tested to check a range of conditions relating to the bones, heart, nerves and kidneys. High levels usually indicate issues with your parathyroid, which is linked to hormone imbalances.

Inorganic phosphate: Phosphate testing is used to help assess the presence of diseases that affect the digestive system, and can interfere with the absorption of phosphate, calcium and magnesium. It can also be an indicator that there are problems with the kidneys.

Uric acid: This is an indicator of high sugar levels and fructose malabsorption. The range should be 266–474umol/L. A low uric acid result may indicate a deficiency of B12, copper or molybdenum.

Action plan

➜ **Drink, drink and then drink some more:** But only water! Dehydration is one of the most stressful states for healthy kidneys. Drinking 6–8 glasses of water a day keeps them flushed out and healthy. (See also Chapter 20.)

➜ **Look at your stress:** Kidneys are damaged by emotional stress and closely connected to fear in Traditional Chinese Medicine (TCM) terms. Do you have any memories or fears that are holding you back? Write a list and visit a kinesiologist or EFT therapist to help release them. Your doctor may refer you to a counsellor or psychiatrist. Alternatively book a yoga, meditation or chi kung session and learn how to use your breath to control stress (see Chapter 22, page 212).

→ **Get acupuncture:** A session or two of acupuncture can boost your kidney meridian and its pair, the bladder meridian.

TOP TIP

Placing your hands at waist level in the small of your back and leaving them there for five minutes, twice a day for a week, can help re-energize your kidneys.

→ **Try a far-infrared sauna:** This warms the body from within and can reboot the kidneys. The heat helps to expand the capillaries and so improve oxygen levels, blood flow and circulation.

→ **Cut down on salt and sugar:** Both contribute to high blood pressure and blood sugar readings, which can overload your kidneys.

→ **Increase your magnesium levels:** If there is too much calcium in your kidneys and not enough magnesium to dissolve it, you may get kidney stones. Rub magnesium oil into your lower back to boost your kidneys.

→ **Take sodium bicarbonate:** Drinking 600mg of sodium bicarbonate, three times a day for two years,[1] can dramatically slow the progress of chronic kidney disease.

→ **Visit a medical herbalist:** Request a herbal tonic specifically designed to strengthen your kidneys. Chanca piedra, goldenrod, hydrangea root, horsetail, celery root, gravel root, uva-ursi, parsley, dandelion root and marshmallow root are all kidney boosters. Health-food stores usually stock herbal-based kidney cleansing kits.

TOP TIP

For a free, online kidney anxiety test visit calmclinic.com.

Chapter 10

The Thymus:
Your Immune System Manager

*'The right raw materials can... double or triple
the protective power of the immune system.'*

JOEL FUHRMAN

You will find the thymus in the centre of your chest, just above your heart, about 4cm (1½in) below the notch in your sternum. The role of the thymus gland is to pump out white blood cells, effectively acting as an incubator for disease-fighting T-cells.

Your immune system manages every aspect of the day-to-day running of your body and works with the other cells, tissues and organs to protect you from infection. A healthy immune system should be able to prevent viruses, bacteria, fungi and parasites from invading your body, and destroy any cells that begin to mutate, as well as rebalance any elements or systems that begin to function less efficiently than they were meant to.

In a nutshell, you only get ill if your immunity is compromised in some way or it malfunctions. For instance, if you suffer from an autoimmune disease where the body attacks its own tissues, you will need your thymus to defend against your own immune system, so it's particularly important to keep it strong and healthy.

Your thymus gland is at its largest in childhood and starts shrinking after puberty. By the time you're in your fifties, you'll have 15 per cent of your thymus left and by the time you get to your early 70s, it will have turned to fatty tissue and vanished entirely. Is the disappearance of your thymus linked to ageing? The question currently being asked in the world of medical research is whether or not rebooting the thymus can reverse the signs of old age. Science, as yet, has no definitive answer, but a current research project is giving thymic hormones to animals in the hope of reversing deterioration.[1]

There are no standard thymus tests, but if you're past the age of 30, your thymus is likely to be in decline. And if you have a hectic, stressful life, its rate of decline may increase. The thymus is the most likely of all your organs to be overwhelmed during stressful times, so it's important to keep it strong and functioning – and particularly if you find yourself succumbing to colds and flu more often than you used to. The thymus is the gateway to your immune system.

Action plan

➜ **Schedule a regular morning thymus tap:** The thymus is said to regulate the energy flow throughout your body. When that energy is low, tapping gently directly above the gland can re-energize and boost your immune system. Tapping the point on your chest over your thymus with the four fingers of your right hand for about 20 seconds daily will keep it awake and working.

➔ **Add in daily supplements:** The following supplements support your thymus and boost your immune system:

- ~ Echinacea, rosehip, olive leaf and yarrow flower essence all serve to strengthen the thymus.

- ~ Antioxidants fight free radicals that can attack the thymus, so also include vitamins C and E.

- ~ Thyme, Pau d'Arco and wheatgrass all support the thymus, as does blackcurrant oil, organic germanium and zinc in combination with vitamin A and beta-carotene.

➔ **Eat foods containing glucosinolates:** These strengthen your thymus, so include plenty of broccoli, cabbage and cauliflower in your diet.

➔ **Try a yoga pose:** Specific poses can stimulate the thymus, so if your immune system needs more support then book a one-to-one appointment with a qualified yoga teacher to work out a programme specifically tailored to your needs.

➔ **Exercise:** Being active increases the blood flow to your thymus, making sure that toxins are released and nutrients can reach the gland.

Chapter 11

The Spleen:
Your Immune System Support

'Above all things physical, it is more important to
be beautiful on the inside – to have a big heart
and an open mind and a spectacular spleen.'

ELLEN DEGENERES

The spleen is located behind the lower ribs on the left-hand side of your tummy above the stomach. It is dark red and about the size of a clenched fist. The spleen has many roles in the immune system, and its main job is to clean up any less than perfect red blood cells and make healthy new white blood cells. It is in charge of filtering your lymph fluid and making antibodies to guard against infection. The spleen also helps fight the bacteria that cause pneumonia and meningitis. It is one of the few organs that can regenerate if it gets damaged and you can live without it if it needs to be surgically removed.

Infection or injury and diseases such as cirrhosis, leukaemia or rheumatoid arthritis can cause your spleen to become swollen and enlarged.

DIAGNOSTIC TESTS

✚ *Doctor*

Your doctor can examine you physically and carry out diagnostic blood tests, CT scans or MRI scans to confirm diagnosis if they think there is a problem. If your spleen is healthy you won't notice it at all, but if it increases in size it can press on your stomach and cause the following symptoms:

- Feeling full very quickly after eating

- Discomfort or pain behind your left ribs

- Anaemia and/or fatigue

- Frequent infections

- Unusual bruising and bleeding

TOP TIP

In Traditional Chinese Medicine (TCM) the spleen is paired with the stomach meridian and, along with digestion, is in charge of taking in, regulating and processing information from the world we live in. With the technology overload of modern life and with TVs, computers, smart phones and other devices bombarding our senses on every side, we all suffer with overstressed spleens from a TCM perspective.

Action plan

➔ **Stress-reduction techniques:** Start meditating or deep breathing to reduce stress. Trauma and repeated chronic stress has been shown to build up excess white blood cells in the spleen, resulting in symptoms of long-term chronic anxiety.[1]

→ **Drink warming teas throughout the day:** Jasmine, raspberry leaf, green tea and chai tea are thought to strengthen the spleen.

→ **Cut down on technology:** Reduce how much time you spend at the computer or on your phone and give your spleen a rest.

→ **Consult a Chinese medical herbalist for a spleen-boosting tonic:** TCM believes that spleen problems stem from a lack of nutrients and from emotional trauma. Any prolapse of an organ may be connected to a deficiency in the spleen energy, and may also be connected to the ability to think clearly and concentrate. The right prescription of medicinal herbs, alongside working on releasing anxiety, can bring the spleen back into balance.

→ **Supplement with spleen-boosting nutrients:** The following supplements can be helpful in strengthening and supporting your spleen:

  ~ Astragalus

  ~ Milk thistle

  ~ Apple cider vinegar capsules (to calm an enlarged spleen) or apple cider vinegar diluted in warm water

  ~ Ginseng

→ **Try acupuncture:** A trained acupuncturist can give you a series of sessions of moxibustion, which is a method of burning herbs above the skin to stimulate the chi, or energy, of your body. The heat warms the cold, stagnant areas that have little energy and gets the spleen energy flowing again. Moxa sticks are also available on the Internet. Google the points appropriate for the spleen and warm the points yourself.

Chapter 12

The Thyroid Gland:
Your Hormone Production
and Control

'Our bodies are finely tuned machines, and if our hormone mixtures aren't "just right", everything goes into disrepair.'

SUZANNE SOMERS

Shaped like a butterfly, the thyroid sits in the middle of your neck, under your chin, and produces hormones that regulate your body temperature, weight and digestion. It also keeps your brain working clearly.

The thyroid makes three important hormones: thyroxine (T4), triiodothyronine (T3) and calcitonin. T3 and T4 are the hormones responsible for your overall metabolism and affect almost every cell in your body. Calcitonin helps regulate calcium stores in the body and the bone-building process.

Thyroid problems are thought to affect up to 50 per cent of us,[1] so it's vital to check how yours is working. Although there is no official medical research on the subject, if your life is stressful, and particularly if you have had a major trauma or shock recently, your thyroid may have stopped working properly. Whiplash from a car accident is also anecdotally linked with low thyroid function. If you have gained or lost weight recently, are always tired, or have been more uptight and frenetic than usual, and notice feeling cold much more than you used to, then it may well be down to your thyroid.

The thyroid gland regulates metabolism: the way your body converts the food you eat into the energy you use to get through the day (moving, thinking and feeling). The hormones secreted by your thyroid gland adjust temperature and brain function as well. If your thyroid isn't working properly, you may feel cold and tired and have high cholesterol levels.

A low, or hypothyroid, condition means that not enough oxygen is getting to your brain. Symptoms include exhaustion, lethargy, depression and feeling cold. Puffiness, hair loss, poor memory, low libido, and muscle and joint aches are common symptoms. A swollen tongue, with rippled 'scalloped' indentations along the sides, is another sign that you may have a low thyroid problem.

On the flipside, an overactive thyroid means that your body temperature will be higher than average. It causes your body and brain to race, and you may have excessive levels of physical and mental energy. Mental and behavioural instability are common, along with weight loss, sweating and anxiety.

TEMPERATURE TEST

 Home

One of the simplest ways to test your thyroid, before consulting your doctor who might then offer you a blood test, is to do a temperature test. Female readers: beware of your monthly menstrual cycle. Don't take your temperature during those few days or you will get an unnaturally high result, as your temperature changes during ovulation. Start the test about three days or so after your period.

1. As soon as you wake up in the morning, before you get out of bed, place a thermometer in your armpit (not under your tongue). The underarm temperature is lower than that measured under the tongue.

2. Leave it there, without moving, for 10 minutes. Make a note of the reading on the chart below.

3. Mark your temperature over a period of days. A pattern should emerge.

ºC															ºF
37.2															99.0
37.1															98.8
37.0															98.6
36.9															98.4
36.8															98.2
36.7															98.0
36.6															97.8
36.5															97.6
36.4															97.4
36.3															97.2
36.2															97.0
36.1															96.8
36.0															96.6
35.9															96.4
35.8															96.2
35.7															96.0
35.6															95.8
Day	1	2	3	4	5	6	7	8	9	10	11	12	13	14	

Sample temperature chart

Understanding your results

Ideally, your readings should lie within the two dark lines. If your temperature is consistently lower than 36.6°C (97.8°F) degrees, or higher than 36.8°C (98.2°F), you may need thyroid support.

BLOOD TEST

✚ *Doctor*

Your doctor can carry out a blood test, but be aware that they are not always reliable. Sometimes the results will be in the normal range, even if you have all the symptoms of a thyroid issue, and your doctor may tell you there is no problem according to those markers. Checking your own temperature, as shown above, and showing the chart to your GP will often help you get treated successfully. Blood tests will establish your levels of TSH (thyroid-stimulating hormone), free thyroxine (free T4) and free T3. You can also ask for your antibody levels to be checked.

Understanding your results

T4: This makes up about 80 per cent of the thyroid's hormones (T3 about 15 per cent). Your body, however, cannot use T4 and has to convert it first to the much more useable T3.

TSH: This hormone is produced by the pituitary gland in the brain and stimulates the thyroid gland into making more. TSH is high when the thyroid is struggling. If you are supplementing and your TSH is low, you are taking too much and should reduce the dosage with your doctor's advice.

Free thyroxine: This is the amount of T4 that is available and not bound to proteins. This reading lowers when the thyroid is struggling.

Free T3: This test measures the total amount of 'free' T3 (i.e. not bound to any other molecules) immediately available. T4 converts to T3 and this is the only thyroid hormone that is actually used by the body's cells. This test is not always offered routinely, but it's worth asking for it, because it will often show low if you are not converting T4 to T3 correctly or high if you have blocked receptor cells.

Antibodies: You can ask your doctor to check your antibody levels. These may be attacking the thyroid and are present if there is a thyroid autoimmune issue. The two most common forms are Hashimoto's disease, where the thyroid is slowly destroyed by the body's own defence system, causing underactivity, and Graves' disease, where the antibodies make the thyroid overactive.

Iodine

Your thyroid needs iodine to work properly. Deficiency is the most common cause of hypothyroidism. If you need to supplement, buy iodine directly from your local health store, as other forms of iodine are toxic for humans. It is hard to overdose, but make sure you follow the instructions on the bottle and dilute it in water if taken orally. Keep neat iodine away from your eyes.

IODINE DEFICIENCY TEST

🏠 *Home*

> Drop three drops of liquid iodine onto the crook of your elbow, rub into a largish bright yellow circle and watch to see how fast the skin sucks it up. If it's still visible by the end of the day, your levels are fine. If it has all vanished within an hour, you need to supplement daily, eat more seaweed and seafood or use iodized salt.

If you are diagnosed as hypothyroid, with an underactive thyroid, your doctor is likely to put you on a prescription for synthetic thyroxine (Levothyroxine). This will reduce your symptoms rapidly but is something you will usually have to take for the rest of your life. You must return for regular blood tests and your doctor will manage your prescription dosage accordingly.

If you have been diagnosed as hyperthyroid, with an overactive thyroid, your doctor will probably prescribe Thioamide, Carbimazole and Propylthiouracil, for instance, which stop your thyroid producing excess hormones. Radioiodine treatment is an alternative, where radiation is used to damage your thyroid, again reducing the hormones produced. Occasionally, surgery is recommended to remove part or all of your thyroid gland and then you will need to take thyroxine for the rest of your life.

Action plan

→ **Go gluten-free if you have Hashimoto's thyroiditis:** Eating gluten, which has nearly the same molecular composition as thyroid tissue, can trigger a mistaken-identity response from your body, so cut it out entirely.

➜ **Check for dairy allergy:** Dairy proteins may cause a reaction with the thyroid gland. If you have Hashimoto's, cutting it out can reduce both your symptoms and your antibody numbers.

➜ **Check for food allergies:** You can consult a nutritionist or go online and order a test kit. Certain foods can cause inflammation and be seen as invaders. Your autoimmune response then springs into action and ends up attacking your organs, your thyroid included.

➜ **Acupuncture:** This has been shown to reduce antibody levels over a series of treatments.[2]

➜ **Adapt your eating habits:** Kale, broccoli, cabbage, cauliflower, spinach, strawberries, peanuts and soya are all goitrogens, which can affect how well your thyroid functions, so only eat small quantities.

➜ **Hair mineral analysis test:** If you think that radiation or toxic metals may have affected you, ask a nutritionist for a test. Heavy metals can weaken your thyroid. Mercury from amalgam dental fillings can be a problem, as can excess copper, arsenic, cadmium and lead. Take chlorella to get them out of your system – it's a slow but thorough treatment. Supplement daily for a year and then test again (see Chapter 24, page 233).

➜ **Detox your environment:** Bromine, fluoride, nitrates in fertilizers and chlorine can all deplete the thyroid gland. Remove them from your environment as much as possible by switching to natural household cleaners, eating organic foods and filtering your water. (See also Chapter 24.)

→ **Get a hormone test:** Stress can elevate your cortisol levels, and too many carbohydrates combined with too few healthy fats can raise your oestrogen levels and throw your thyroid off balance. If your thyroid is struggling, your adrenals are likely to be struggling, too. Balance one and you strengthen the other. (See also Chapter 13.)

→ **Supplement with liposomal glutathione:** A powerful antioxidant that can heal damaged thyroid tissue and fend off attacks from your autoimmune system – and essential if you have Hashimoto's. A naturopathic doctor or nutritionist can advise you.

→ **Boost your thyroid function with natural remedies:**

- For an underactive thyroid, take kelp, calcium and amino acids (tyrosine, glutamine and glycine). Also, ginseng, ginkgo biloba and gotu kola boost energy levels.

- For an overactive thyroid, lycopus may help with palpitations and shaking, and motherwort with palpitations and tachycardia.

→ **Up your minerals and vitamins too:**

- Vitamin A to convert T4 to T3.

- Vitamin B1 for an overactive thyroid.

- Vitamin B2 for thyroid hormone production.

- Vitamin B6 to help make thyroid hormones.

- Vitamin B12 cannot be absorbed properly if you have an underactive thyroid and deficiency is associated with mental health issues.

- Vitamins C and E help control and balance thyroid hormone production.

- Magnesium, zinc and selenium help conversion of T4 to T3.

Chapter 13

The Adrenals:
Your Stress Controllers

*'The natural healing force in each one of us
is the greatest force in getting well.'*

HIPPOCRATES

The adrenals are part of your body's endocrine or hormone-producing system. These two tiny glands (the right one is triangular and the left shaped more like a half-moon) sit on top of your kidneys. Each adrenal gland has two distinct parts: the outer adrenal cortex and the inner medulla, both of which produce different types of hormones and are responsible for regulating many of the body's functions, including creating energy by converting carbohydrates, proteins and fats into blood glucose, maintaining the electrolyte balance in the body's fluids and fat storage.

The adrenal cortex produces aldosterone, cortisol and androgens (progesterone, oestrogen and testosterone). Inside is the adrenal medulla, and the chromaffin cells of the medulla are the body's main source of catecholamines: adrenaline and noradrenaline.

Cortisol, in particular, is important in balancing the body's systems and is released along with adrenaline as part of the body's 'fight or flight' response. This primal physiological system was designed to protect us from genuine threats to life, such as wild animals or in battle. The release of adrenaline diverts blood away from the brain and stomach, and sends it instead to the muscles to either fight off or flee the threat.

The problem with modern life is that many of us experience this response on a daily basis. An unexpected bill, being stuck in traffic, a stressful exchange or an e-mail at work, or your toddler throwing a tantrum can all trigger 'flight or fight', even though there is no actual threat to life. And experiencing regular high levels of stress (or high levels of cortisol) over a long period of time can overwhelm your adrenals. Continually working, they get exhausted by the constant demand and eventually stop functioning properly. Signs that you're heading towards burnout can include:

- Fatigue

- Craving sugary and fatty foods

- Mood swings and depressed mood

- Dry skin and hair loss

- Inability to handle stress

In today's super-stressful world, when so many of us are frantically trying to balance competing demands on our time and feel as if we're playing constant catch-up, our 'fight or flight' system is switched on constantly.[1] A high level of cortisol and adrenaline becomes habitual and none of it is good for us.

Cushing's syndrome and Addison's disease are two serious adrenal disorders. Cushing's syndrome is the result of too much cortisol, and Addison's disease is the result of too little cortisol and damage to the adrenals.

WHITE LINE TEST

 Home

This simple test will help you check if your adrenals are seriously drained (although it doesn't work so well for just slight adrenal fatigue).

With your fingernail, draw a sharp line across your bare stomach or on your inner forearm. If your adrenals are working well, the line will turn white then red within 15 to 20 seconds.

If the line turns red more rapidly that may indicate excessive adrenal activity. When your adrenals are struggling, however, your blood pressure tends to lower, with the blood vessels widening as a result. Light stimulation of the skin in this case will cause those blood vessels to contract and narrow, whitening the skin instead.

So if the line stays white and gets wider after a few minutes, then you may have a problem. This is an indicator test only and should be followed up by a consultation with your doctor.

SALIVA TEST

🏠 *Home* ✚ *Doctor*

The most reliable way to measure your levels of cortisol is with a saliva test, where samples are taken four times in a 24-hour period. This will analyse the levels of cortisol in your system and identify how your adrenals are functioning.

Genova Diagnostics (gdx.net) is a reputable UK company offering a wide range of diagnostic tests. Biolab Medical Unit (biolab.co.uk) offers similar services. Their tests can only be accessed via a doctor or a nutritionist. It is a good idea to book a consultation with a nutritionist, who will send you the appropriate kit and then meet with you, or discuss the results over the phone, and can then offer guidance regarding nutritional rebalancing for any issues.

BLOOD TEST FOR CORTISOL

✚ *Doctor*

Ask your GP for a standard blood test for cortisol (has to be done within an hour of waking up in the morning). The reference range UG/DL is usually 4–20, but for optimal health it should be 10–15. See zrtlab.com for an example test result.

Action plan

→ **Reduce stress:** Take time to have a good look at your lifestyle and make changes to reduce your stress levels. Long-term stress can burn you out, so it is vital to reduce your load. Write a list of everything that stresses you and how best you can resolve the issues. Don't expect an immediate recovery either, as your adrenals can take a year or more to reinvigorate. Rest is the ultimate answer. Keep at it and keep monitoring your adrenals with the home test. (See also Chapter 22.)

→ **Deep breathing:** This calms the mind and can turn off that 'fight or flight' switch by persuading it that there is no danger nearby. Take five minutes each day to lie down quietly and use diaphragmatic breathing (see Chapter 22, page 212). You might also like to close your eyes, bring your adrenals to mind and picture them lying on a sunbed in their sunshades, glass of fresh juice in hand on a beach in the sun somewhere. That's the chilled energy they need to experience to recover – and it doesn't happen overnight.

→ **Pay attention to your diet:** Avoid sugars, caffeine, hydrogenated oils and processed foods that may further drain your adrenals. Add in green leafy vegetables for magnesium and other nutrients.

→ **Do food allergy tests:** Cut out any foods that you are sensitive to. When your body is allergic to something, it releases histamine and other inflammatory substances. Your body is then forced to release large amounts of cortisol to calm the inflammation down, draining your already exhausted adrenals still further. Remove the allergy and you break the cycle and give your adrenals a chance to recover. (See also Chapter 18.)

→ **Sort your sleep:** Make sure you get plenty of rest and aim to get to bed before 11 p.m. each night when a second cortisol surge (that will exhaust your adrenals unnecessarily) often happens. (See also Chapter 23.)

→ **Supplement daily:**

~ Vitamin B5 helps the adrenals produce sex and stress hormones.

~ B6 is also involved in creating adrenal hormones.

~ B12 deficiency is linked to adrenal cortex stress.

~ B12 and folic acid will boost your energy levels.

~ Selenium: Low levels of selenium are also linked to adrenal issues.

→ **Add adrenal supporting herbs:** Naturopaths or herbalists can usually advise and provide you with an invigorating tonic. In particular:

~ Ashwagandha, one of nature's superfoods, is known to combat adrenal fatigue by lowering cortisol levels.

~ Rhodiola, holy basil, liquorice root and ginseng can all help your body to adapt to stress and boost your energy levels.

→ **Watch for symptoms:** Dehydration and electrolyte depletion are often symptoms of adrenal fatigue. Drink water. Rehydrate your cells. If it doesn't seem to work and you are craving salt and often thirsty, visit your medical practitioner and ask them to check you for adrenal fatigue and to monitor your aldosterone levels.

➜ **Check:** Regularly check your standard medical prescriptions with your doctor, as overuse of pharmaceutical drugs may make your adrenal exhaustion worse.

➜ **Iodine deficiency:** There is often a connection between low iodine levels, and thyroid function and adrenal stress, so test your iodine levels and supplement if necessary (see Chapter 12, page 106).

Chapter 14

The Blood:
Your Vital Force

*'Today, blood work and science are able to provide
more of a movie of your health, identifying
trends before they become an issue.'*

Elizabeth Holmes

Your blood accounts for 7 per cent of your body weight; it is your life force and nothing in your body would work without it. Part of the circulatory system, along with the lymphatic system (which we'll look at in the following chapter), your blood carries vital nutrients and hormones, along with oxygen, through your arteries to every far-flung corner of your body, and takes away waste products and carbon dioxide on its return trip via your veins. Each and every day your blood travels through more than 125,000km (80,000 miles) of capillaries, veins and arteries. It cools your liver, heart, muscles and brain, making sure they don't overheat. And at the same time moves that heat to your fingers and toes, keeping them warm, when logically they should be very cold indeed.

Plasma is the clear, pale liquid that carries the many types of red and white blood cells and platelets that make up your blood. It also contains more than 700 proteins that are used to help your body function.

Red blood cells get their distinctive colour from haemoglobin, a chemical that contains iron. The cells carry oxygen and collect carbon dioxide, taking it to the lungs to be breathed out. If, for some reason, your red blood cells get sick, you will feel extremely tired and are likely to be diagnosed with anaemia.

Anaemia is usually due to lack of iron and this may be triggered by more serious health problems, including bleeding or inflammation in your gut, stomach ulcers, kidney disease, heavy periods, stomach or bowel cancer. Your bone marrow needs iron to make haemoglobin for your red blood cells.

Your white blood cells attack and fend off the bacteria and viruses that are continually trying to invade your body. Each millilitre of your blood has around 5,000–7,000 white blood cells, working with your antibodies to give you immunity against disease.

The platelets are like tiny sticking plasters, circulating round your body in your blood until they find some sort of damage in a blood vessel, such as a cut or wound, and then form a clot that stops the flow of blood.

BLOOD TEST

✚ *Doctor*

Doctors usually order blood tests to find out what's going on with you when you have any sort of health problem. You may well have had extensive tests carried out in the past, but it's important to get a copy of the results and ask your doctor to go through them with you.

Understanding your results

Usually, there is a reference range in a column on the far-right side of the page, giving normal healthy readings. In a middle column, you will find your own result, which you can compare to the reference ranges. If it is higher or lower than normal, it may be printed in bold, or will have an 'H' for high, or 'L' for low by its side to flag that there is an issue.

Ask what each one means for you and whether or not your doctor considers the standard range (the readings given) reliable. Then ask for their suggestions as to how to bring any levels that have shown up too high or too low back to within the normal result range. Take notes so you don't forget. Don't worry if you find your levels are high in many of the tests. With a few simple steps, you can turn yourself around in a matter of weeks.

Different countries use different figures to determine the health of their citizens. UK and USA blood test numbers are different and so are their ranges – the low to high numbers that define low to high 'normal'. Whatever the numbers used, all you are interested in is where your result sits in comparison to the numbers judged by the doctors of different lands to be those of a healthy individual.

The first section of your blood test will be headed 'haematology' and this is a series of individual tests that give a comprehensive overview of the health or otherwise of your blood. The following explains what it means:

Haemoglobin: Haemoglobin is a protein molecule in red blood cells that carries oxygen from the lungs to your tissues and cells. If your haemoglobin levels are low, you are likely to be diagnosed with anaemia, a condition in which your body is not getting enough oxygen, causing exhaustion and general weakness. If your haemoglobin levels are high, this usually means you have too many red cells. This can eventually cause the blood to become too thick, potentially leading to heart problems or strokes.

Haematocrit: Haematocrit measures the amount of space red blood cells take up in the blood. It is reported as a percentage (0–100) or a proportion (0–1).

RBC: Red blood cell count analyses the actual number of red blood cells per volume of blood. Both increases and decreases in numbers can indicate a problem. Decreased numbers point to anaemia; increased numbers to an excess of production, or to fluid loss due to diarrhoea, dehydration or burns.

MCV: Mean corpuscular volume is a measurement of the average size of your red blood cells. The MCV is elevated when your RBCs are larger than normal, for example in anaemia caused by vitamin B12 deficiency or folic acid deficiency; or if there is a problem with your liver, you have an underactive thyroid or are pregnant. When the MCV is decreased, your RBCs are smaller than normal, which may indicate iron deficiency anaemia or inflammation.

MCH: Mean corpuscular haemoglobin (MCH) is a calculation of the amount of oxygen-carrying haemoglobin inside your RBCs.

RDW: Red cell distribution width is a calculation of the variation in the size of your RBCs. Increased RDW indicates an abnormal variation in RBC size. It can also indicate iron, B12 or folic acid deficiency or bone marrow disorders.

Platelets: The platelet count is the number of platelets in a given volume of blood. Both increases and decreases can point to bleeding or bone marrow disorders. Increased numbers of platelets occur after bleeding, inflammation, infection and surgery, in bone marrow disorders and in patients with absent or underactive spleens. Decreased numbers are associated with immune conditions, vitamin deficiencies, some drugs (especially chemotherapy), alcoholism, liver disease, enlarged spleen, bone marrow disorders and some rare inherited disorders.

MPV: Mean platelet volume (MPV) is a machine-calculated measurement of the average size of your platelets. New platelets are larger and an increased MPV occurs when increased numbers of platelets are being produced. Younger platelets are larger than older ones.

WBC: This is a count of the actual number of white blood cells per volume of blood. Increases can be caused by infections, inflammation and sometimes cancer or leukaemia; decreases can be caused by pharmaceutical drugs or may indicate an autoimmune problem. Viruses, severe infections, bone marrow failure, an enlarged spleen, liver disease and alcohol excess can also cause levels to lower.

There are five different types of white blood cell, each with its own function in protecting us from infection: neutrophils, lymphocytes, monocytes, eosinophils and basophils.

1. **Neutrophils:** Neutrophils are one of the first lines of defence against bacterial infection. Levels change from day to day depending on what is going on in your body.

The 'normal' level of neutrophils differs between ethnic groups.

2. **Lymphocytes:** These often increase or decrease if you have a viral infection.

3. **Monocytes:** These often increase when there is some type of infection such as tuberculosis or a bone marrow disorder.

4. **Eosinophils:** Numbers may increase because of asthma, hay fever, eczema, drug allergies and parasitic infections.

5. **Basophils:** Can be increased because of infections, inflammatory disorders or bone marrow disorders, e.g. chronic myeloid leukaemia.

ESR: Erythrocyte sedimentation rate – an indicator of how much your cells are clumping. When you have healthy, happy cells they float freely and separately. If there is inflammation or an infection, the cells will clump together in sticky groups. When your ESR result is above 10 it's not good – under 10 is a healthy reading.

Sodium: Sodium is an electrolyte that is found in all body fluids. It regulates the amount of water in the body, controlling blood pressure in the process. Symptoms of a possible problem include dehydration, swelling or blood pressure problems.

Potassium: Like sodium, potassium is present in all body fluids, but mainly within your cells, with only a very small amount in the serum or plasma component of the blood. If potassium levels rise or fall, it can affect your muscles and your nerves. It may also point to either a high blood pressure problem or an issue with your kidneys.

TESTING FOR IRON

✚ *Doctor*

Serum Iron: This tests whether or not your iron levels are normal. If you don't take in enough iron from your food, then your iron levels drop, which can trigger anaemia. Absorption of too much iron, however, causes excessive build-up of iron in the tissues, damaging your heart, liver or pancreas.

UIBC: Tests whether your iron stores are too high or too low.

Ferritin: The ferritin concentration within your bloodstream reflects the amount of iron stored in your body.

TIBC: Stands for total iron-binding capacity. Readings show the ability of your blood to bind and transport iron, giving a good picture of your overall iron stores.

Your blood test will give you a clear picture of what is going on in your body and where follow-up is required. Follow the instructions in the appropriate chapters of this book to support whichever organ is struggling. Go back to your doctor for repeat tests at regular intervals to monitor your progress.

Action plan

→ **Diet, exercise and stress reduction:** These are the lifestyle choices that can improve and reverse blood numbers in a relatively short period of time. Change your patterns and you can change your blood at a cellular level. You'll find more help in the following chapters:

- ~ For healthy eating see Chapter 19.

- ~ To get the lowdown on exercise, see Chapter 20.

- ~ To address the impact of stress, see Chapter 22.

Hypoglycaemia

Non-diabetic hypoglycaemia is a condition that causes blood glucose levels to drop too low. In its extreme form it is relatively rare, but many people who aren't officially hypoglycaemic still suffer from blood sugar swings if they are including too many carbohydrates and unhealthy foods in their diet. Common symptoms include shakiness and fatigue, increased appetite, dizziness and irritability. White flour, rice, potatoes, cakes and biscuits all turn rapidly into sugar and artificially spike your energy levels, causing you to feel great initially but then falling off in equivalently low drops that can make you feel extremely ill.

Use the following three tests for hypoglycaemia and be reassured that it is totally reversible if you make a few lifestyle changes.

GLUCOSE TEST

✚ *Doctor*

In order to establish whether or not you suffer from hypoglycaemia, a doctor will need to test your blood glucose at regular intervals. A blood glucose test looks like a mountain range with deep valleys, the ups and downs reflecting the timings of the peaks and troughs of your blood sugar swings. If you feel like you have fallen off a cliff every afternoon at 5 p.m., then a deep low on your test shows you why.

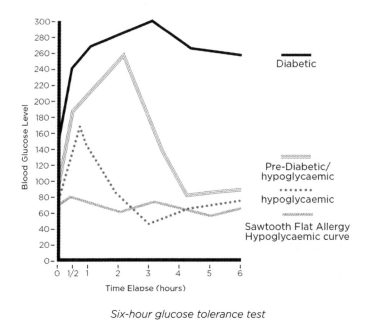

Six-hour glucose tolerance test

URINE TEST

🏠 *Home*

A saline refractometer is a handy tool to keep an eye on your blood sugar levels, particularly if you are suffering from mood swings due to hypoglycaemia or are prediabetic and wanting to reverse the condition before it develops into something more serious. A refractometer reads salt levels in your urine, which mimics your blood sugar levels.

A normal urine reading is 12–18 on the refractometer. Prediabetic will come in at 55–60 and below 9 will mean you are hypoglycaemic, dehydrated or, again, prediabetic.

SUGAR METER TEST

🏠 *Home*

You can use a blood sugar meter to get readings in between your doctor's regular tests. You can buy these online or in the chemist. You prick your finger with a small, sharp needle, put a drop of blood on a test strip and then put it in a meter that shows your blood sugar level.

Action plan

→ **Avoid certain foods:** Don't eat sugar of any kind – including honey, fruit or juice. Also avoid any foods made with white flour, such as bread, cakes, biscuits, pasta, etc. Substances like caffeine and nicotine can also affect your blood sugar. Nicotine affects your insulin production, causing extra glucose production. Caffeine is a particular problem for people with Type 2 diabetes, as it raises both blood sugar and insulin levels. So, if you have diabetes and need your coffee fix, but want to avoid that blood sugar spike and crash, stick to decaf or green tea. If you decide to cut out caffeine then you are likely to get slight withdrawal symptoms for the first couple of weeks, including headaches and feeling moody or emotional and tired. Persevere, as these symptoms disappear after 10 days or so and you'll feel much better with steady blood sugar levels.

→ **Eat more nuts:** These contain healthy fats that slow the absorption of sugar. Stick to a small handful a day, as nuts are full of protein, fibre, vitamins, minerals and heart-healthy fats, but they are also high in calories.

➜ **Eat more fibre:** Oats, bran, barley and rye contain beta-glucan that stops your blood sugar spiking.

➜ **Cut back on alcohol and never drink on an empty stomach:** Different drinks contain different amounts of sugar – beer, cider, sherry, alcopops and lager will initially raise your blood glucose and then later cause it to plunge, increasing your risk of hypoglycaemia. No more than 14 units a week, the equivalent of 6 pints of beer or 10 small glasses of wine, are generally recommended, but if you have blood sugar issues, there is no safe amount of alcohol. Try to restrict yourself to low-alcohol drinks and be aware that alcohol can make hypoglycaemic medications less effective.

➜ **Eat your greens:** A diet high in green leafy vegetables can also prevent blood sugar surges.

➜ **Apple cider vinegar:** This slows sugar absorption and can be taken (2 tablespoons) before meals.

➜ **Cinnamon:** This has been shown to drop fasting blood sugar levels significantly. In one research study, it was found that taking between a half and three teaspoons of cinnamon daily over 40 days cut blood sugar levels by 24 per cent.[1-2]

➜ **Supplement to help stabilize blood sugar levels:** Bio recovery (bio-recoveryinc.com) have a full hypoglycaemia supplement package that contains the correct balance of the following:

~ Vitamin C

~ Vitamin B complex

~ Niacin

- ~ Pantothenic acid

- ~ Potassium

- ~ Manganese

- ~ Chromium

- ~ Glutamine

Chapter 15

The Lymph:
Your Waste Removal System

'Move your lymph system. Lymph is like a sewage system that carries all of the toxins out of your body.'

VALENTINA ZELYAEVA

Along with blood, the lymphatic system forms part of the circulatory system, but it also has an important role to play in your immune system. Lymph is very similar to blood plasma in that it contains lymphocytes and waste products, and prevents the body from being overwhelmed by toxins, bacteria and cancerous cells.

Your body is covered by a delicate, intricate network of lymph capillaries; 70 per cent of these lie just under the top layer of your skin, carrying a clear liquid that drains toxins and excess fluid from your tissues in the same way that veins carry blood around the body. Lymph is where many of the lymphocytes, the white blood cells, live, and their job is to destroy abnormal cells and fight infections. If your lymph is working properly, it's hard for disease to get a foothold. It's therefore vital to keep it flowing.

Your lymph nodes are found all over the body, with the largest groups in the neck, groin and armpits. The spleen and thymus are also part of this system and act as filters, protective gatekeepers that gather up and destroy any nasties that infiltrate your lymph fluid. A thoroughly efficient defence system, they catch the invaders, wipe out bacteria and break down cancer cells.

If you find a pea-sized lump in any of the areas marked in the illustration below, your immune system may be struggling to filter efficiently and it's time to take action yourself. The nodes can swell and get painful if they are infected.

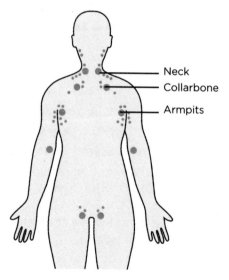

Neck
Collarbone
Armpits

Location of lymph nodes

Lymphoedema is a long-term problem that results from a blockage somewhere in the lymphatic network, causing substantial swelling and discomfort. Sometimes this can happen as a result of an injury or infection, or after surgery where the nodes are removed. If you catch lymphoedema early, the swelling can be managed and held in check. Book an appointment with your doctor, too, to check there is nothing serious going on.

LYMPH CHECK

 Home

Join your three first fingers together and gently press each area of the lymph nodes (see illustration opposite). If any area feels hard and slightly swollen or you can feel a small lump that's a bit sore, then you may have an infection. Usually this will disappear after a few days, but sometimes it can be an indicator of more serious issues, so always get any lump immediately checked out by your doctor – even if you have had one before.

Action plan

→ **Exercise:** Dancing, walking, jumping – any movement stimulates the lymph to flush out toxins. (See also Chapter 20.)

TOP TIP

If you prefer to exercise at home, then 20 minutes' daily rebounding may well be the one for you. This exercise not only tones your body and boosts your energy, but is also the most effective way of activating your lymph. Anecdotal reports suggest that even five minutes of bouncing daily can reduce the size of cysts and lumps, and sometimes make them vanish entirely. Well worth a try! The Bellicon rebounder is the best I have found (bellicon.com).

→ **Dry skin brushing:** Invest in a dry skin brush and stimulate your lymph just before you shower. Before you turn on the tap, move the brush several times from the tips of your limbs towards your heart, brushing firmly enough to feel slightly uncomfortable. Work thoroughly, front and back from top to toe. Always brush towards the heart.

→ **Manual lymphatic drainage massage:** Done with a feather-light touch, this is one of the most relaxing ways of getting your lymph moving. Experiment until you find a therapist who works for you.

→ **Try a warm compress with apple cider vinegar:** This can reduce the swelling in the lymph glands, increasing blood circulation and helping with pain. Leave the compress in place for five minutes before patting dry.

TOP TIP

Rubbing colloidal silver onto the infected lymph node may help. Colloidal silver is antibacterial, antiviral and antifungal so can hit most infections on the head, rapidly and effectively. Usually, after two to three days of a twice-daily application, the lump disappears. If it doesn't, consult your doctor immediately for further testing.

→ **Increase your water intake:** The lymphatic system is made up primarily of water, so it's important to keep yourself hydrated by drinking plenty of water. (See also Chapter 20.)

Chapter 16

The Skeleton:
Your Structural Support

'Research clearly shows us that the earlier women think about maintaining their bone mass and take steps to do so, the better their health will be in the long run.'

Lois Capps

You probably take your bones for granted. Most of us do. But as you age, it's vital to keep them strong and healthy. Your skeleton is what keeps you upright and it has six major functions; support, movement, protection, production of blood cells, storage of minerals and endocrine regulation.

An adult has 206 bones, which can be divided into the 'axial skeleton' and the 'appendicular skeleton'. The axial skeleton is formed by the vertebral column, which protects the spinal cord, the ribcage, the skull and other associated bones. The shoulder girdle, the pelvic girdle and the bones of the upper and lower limbs form the appendicular skeleton.

Your bone mass reaches maximum density around age 21, but after 35 the body starts to remove more bone than it replaces.

Your bones don't look any different from the outside but inside, the cortical 'shell' thins and the struts that make up the inner structure become thinner and sometimes break down. As a result, the total amount of bone tissue starts to decrease, which is why we become more vulnerable to fractures and osteoporosis.[1]

There are many risk factors for osteoporosis apart from age. These include your family history, not developing good bone mass when you are young (due to lack of vitamin D) and menopause can also cause bone density to reduce by up to 70 per cent.[2] Having low bone mass doesn't mean you'll get osteoporosis, but the risk increases, and it's important to know how healthy your bones are and take steps to maintain them. Frightening? Check your bone density annually and keep track of what it's doing over time, and you can kick that fear into the long grass.

ACCUDEXA TEST

✚ *Doctor*

> If you are female and are in, or past, menopause, you can presume that your bones have lost mass and are weaker than they used to be. You can request a bone density scan via your medical practitioner, although this test is not usually free.
>
> The AccuDEXA is accurate and has been clinically evaluated. You place your middle finger in a small machine, it scans you and then gives a value that accurately indicates the overall bone density of the rest of the bones in your body. If it is low, don't panic, because correct supplementation and exercise will reboot your bones.

Action plan

→ **Eat more broccoli, cabbage, parsley and onions:** These foods maintain bone health, and can reduce bone mass decline and osteoporosis risk.[3-4]

→ **Eat protein:** Bone is made of 50 per cent protein and the more you eat (about 100g/3½oz a day is ideal), the better your bone density, as long as you also eat vegetables.[5] Protein doesn't have to come purely from meat; other alternatives include hemp, pumpkin or chia seeds, broccoli, tofu, almonds, nuts and teff or amaranth.

→ **Exercise:** Weight-bearing exercises, such as running or weight lifting, can build up your bones and prevent them deteriorating further.[6-7] Vibrating exercise machines have been found to be good, as have body-balancing exercises. Yoga can help, alongside muscle strength training and high-speed interval training.[8]

→ **Take calcium:** This is the most important mineral for healthy bones, but ideally you need to get it from foods rather than supplements. Calcium-rich foods include seeds, sardines, green leafy vegetables, tinned salmon, beans and lentils, almonds and rhubarb. And of course, if you eat dairy, yoghurt and cheeses. Magnesium and zinc-rich foods are key – dark chocolate, avocado and nuts – and omega-3 rich chia, flaxseeds and walnut also help increase bone growth.[8]

→ **Avoid alcohol, fizzy drinks, sugar, processed meats and foods:** All these foods leach calcium from your bones and trigger inflammation. Fizzy drinks contain phosphoric acid and chemicals that cause mineral and bone loss. If you can't resist them, a calcium supplement daily will reduce the effects. Drinking coffee is no longer thought to be a bone-destroying habit – apparently, just 2 tablespoons of added milk negates any harmful effects.

➜ **Supplement:** Include magnesium, calcium citrate and vitamin D3. Vitamin K2 and strontium are also recommended for bone health (see also Chapter 19, page 185 and the Appendix).

➜ **Try essential oils:** Reputed to help with bone repair, try mixing a few drops of *Helichrysum*, Fir or Cypress essential oils with a carrier oil – olive oil, shea butter, refined coconut oil or sweet almond oil work well – and then rub into the skin above the bone three times a day to increase bone density in that area.

Chapter 17

Body Fat:
Your Thermal Insulator

'The simple answer as to why we get fat is that carbohydrates make us so; protein and fat do not.'

GARY TAUBES

Fat is not just a by-product of eating too many biscuits, it is actually a hormone-producing substance that can dramatically disrupt your health, if you have too much of it. There are distinctly different types of fat and some are more dangerous than others.

White fat stores energy and in healthy-weight adults composes 20 per cent of weight in men and 25 per cent weight in women. As well as being our thermal insulator, adipose tissue also produces oestrogen and, if your body fat is too high, that means an increase in your risk of cancer, stroke and Type 2 diabetes.

Brown fat generates body heat and is more like muscle than white fat. Although we have considerably less of it, exercise, cold temperatures and regularly eating small quantities of food can trigger it to burn off the white fat.

Subcutaneous fat sits just under the skin on the arms and legs, thighs and bottom, and produces the hormone leptin, also known as the hunger hormone (see Chapter 19, page 187). It can be accurately measured with callipers that test your total body fat.

Visceral fat is the most dangerous of all and it is linked to being overweight and poor lifestyle choices, such as eating a high-sugar, high-fat diet, smoking and lack of exercise. Some people are more prone to storing fat this way than others. Visceral fat sits inside the abdominal cavity, building up around the liver, kidneys, pancreas and intestines, causing potential problems with high blood pressure, insulin resistance and high cholesterol levels. Visceral fat is also associated with high stress levels and it increases as cortisol levels increase. It disrupts hormones and increases the risk of getting Type 2 diabetes, breast cancer and Alzheimer's.[1]

The four root causes of fat that won't shift despite exercise, diet and supplementation are:

- Slow metabolism, which can be to do with an underactive thyroid.

- Hormonal imbalance due to problems with insulin and oestrogen, progesterone and testosterone hormone levels.

- Raised cortisol levels due to continual and chronic stress from everyday life.

- High level of toxicity – from toxins in your food, water and air, and in the household products you use, many of which mimic and upset hormones.

BODY MASS INDEX (BMI) TEST

🏠 *Home*

Your BMI is a measurement used by doctors and health professionals to judge if your body weight is healthy for your height, gender and age. Although it's a blunt instrument, and for those who are athletic and have a lot of muscle can be misleading, it can offer a useful at-a-glance measure of health. BMI is most often flagged in connection with the dangers of being overweight – but being underweight with a low BMI can be equally dangerous. Not only is it likely to indicate a deficiency of nutrient uptake, but it may also be linked to an inability to absorb vitamins, minerals and amino acids, all essential for optimal health.

To work out your BMI, divide your weight in kilograms by your height in metres and then divide your answer by your height again. This gives your BMI score.

Understanding your results

- 15–16 is severely underweight and less than 15 is very severely underweight

- Under 18.5 is low and considered underweight

- A healthy score is 18.5–24.9

- 25–29.9 is considered overweight

- 30–39.9 is obese

- 40 plus is morbidly obese

If you want to avoid the maths, there are several free BMI calculators on the Internet, which are both quick and easy to use. If you are underweight wanting to gain a few pounds, or overweight and wanting to lose some, keeping an eye on your BMI is an effective way to track your progress.

WAIST-TO-HEIGHT RATIO (WHTR) TEST

🏠 *Home*

This seems to be a more accurate assessment for those who are pear- rather than apple-shaped, or for serious fitness devotees or bodybuilders, and is calculated by dividing the size of your waist by your height. All you need for this is a tape measure.

Understanding your results

A result of less than 0.5 is considered healthy. Greater than 0.5 indicates higher risk of diabetes, heart disease and stroke. The WHO (World Health Organization) assesses the waist circumference only. Men are considered to be at increased risk with a waist size of 94cm (37in) and at substantially increased risk with a waist of 102cm (40in). For women its 80cm (31in) and 88cm (35in) respectively.[2] For each 3–4kg (6–8lb) of weight you lose, you lose a corresponding 2.5cm (1in) from your waistline.

BASAL METABOLIC RATE TEST

🏠 *Home*

Your metabolism can be fast or slow, depending on your age, body size and genes. Men tend to be more muscular, with heavier bones and have less fat than women, and so tend to have a faster metabolism. Your basal metabolic rate (BMR) indicates the number of calories it takes for your body to keep functioning while sitting entirely still. When you know your BMR, you can work out how many calories you should be eating daily to keep a healthy weight. To find out what yours is, check the free BMR calculators online.

Understanding your results

Your BMR decreases as you age. A slow metabolic rate means that you tend to burn food slowly. One of the best reasons for exercising is to up your BMR by building your muscle tone, because muscle tissue burns many more calories than body fat, even while you are resting and doing absolutely nothing. For example, 4.5kg (10lb) of muscle will burn 50 calories in a day spent doing nothing, while 4.5kg (10lb) of fat will burn only 20. Building muscle, doing cardiovascular exercise, walking, going out in the cold or turning off your central heating will all help increase your BMR.

FOOD ANALYSIS TEST

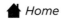 *Home*

This test is designed to make you aware – of whether you are eating less healthily than you think and of any poor eating habits you have.

Answer the following questions:

1. How many times a day do you eat?

> Main meals (times of day)......................................
>
> Snacks (times of day)..

2. How many servings do you eat of:

    Fruit ....

    Vegetables (cooked and raw) ....

    Wholegrains ....

    Protein ....

    Dairy products ....

    Other ....

3. Do you eat:

    Fried foods ....

    Sugar ....

    Margarine ....

    Fast foods ....

    Sweets/candy ....

    Microwaved food ....

    Processed meats ....

    Aspartame/artificial sweeteners ....

    Food cooked in aluminium pans ....

    Refined foods ....

4. How many glasses a day do you drink of:

    Bottled water ....

    Tap water ....

    Milk ....

    Fresh fruit juices ....

Tea ....

Coffee ....

Fruit juices (cartons) ....

Red wine ....

White wine ....

Beer...

Spirits ....

Fresh vegetable juices ....

Herbal tea ....

Fizzy drinks (regular and diet)..

5. How often do you eat meat? Daily, 3–5 times a week or once a week/less?

    ....

6. How often do you eat dairy products? Daily, 3–5 times a week, once a week/less?

    ....

7. What are your favourite foods? How often do you eat them?

    ....

8. Do you avoid certain foods? If so, why?

    ....

9. Do you experience any symptoms if meals are missed?

    ....

10. Do you experience any symptoms after meals?

....

~~~~~~

Action plan

→ **Take regular measurements:** Keep an eye on your visceral fat levels and measure your waist regularly. For an inexpensive monitor, the Tanita scales accurately measure weight, visceral fat, body fat, water content and muscle levels, as well as your base metabolic rate.

→ **Lose weight:** Reducing your calorie intake and increasing your daily exercise is really the only way to lose weight. Aim for slow and steady weight loss through lifestyle changes rather than a crash diet and you'll keep the pounds from returning. (See also Chapters 17 and 19.)

→ **Eat lentils:** They contain inulin, a starchy substance that helps breaks down visceral fat.

→ **Reduce stress:** High cortisol levels and a stressful lifestyle can make you more likely to reach for comfort food and pile on the pounds. Release your issues and watch your body release its weight. (See also Chapter 22.)

→ **Food allergies:** These can slow down weight loss, so try keeping a food diary for a month or so and observe if any of your symptoms flare up after eating or drinking specific foods. You may find a clear pattern. Often, the food you like the best is the one your body tolerates least. Cut it out and see if there is a difference. Make whatever changes work for you. (See also Chapter 18.)

→ **Hot lemon and cayenne:** Starting the day with a glass of hot lemon water with a pinch of cayenne pepper increases thermogenesis, which then boosts metabolism.[3]

→ **Green tea:** Reputed to speed up fat oxidation and raises your metabolic rate.[3] Drink several cups a day or take a 400mg capsule daily.

→ **Oil pulling:** Put one tablespoon of organic coconut oil in your mouth and swish it around your gums for 15 minutes or so to detox your mouth and speed up your metabolism. Don't swallow the oil – just brush your teeth after you have finished.

Chapter 18

The Last Pieces
of the Jigsaw

'Health is the greatest possession.'

LAO TZU

There are various other tests you can do that will give you a clear picture of what is going on in the rest of your body. Together, they will fill in the missing parts of your health jigsaw puzzle.

Cold spots

When one of your organs has a problem, you may notice a cold spot. This is where the sweat glands have stopped working properly.

If, for instance, there is a cold spot on the right side of your body at the base of the diaphragm near the bottom of your ribs, it relates to the gallbladder or the gall duct. On the opposite side, at the bottom of the ribs, a cold spot will relate to problems in the pancreas or spleen. If you have breathing problems, the cold spot will be at the end of the breastbone, over the solar plexus. Cold around your lower back means the kidneys aren't happy; on your tummy, the stomach is struggling.

RE-ENERGIZING COLD SPOTS

🏠 *Home* 🌿 *Remedy*

Run your hands over your body – you will notice that your skin feels warm to the touch in the majority of places, but at certain points there is a noticeable temperature drop.

To re-energize any of these cold spots, rub your hands briskly together until they are hot, then place them gently on top of the cold spot. Using this simple practice for two minutes, twice a day, will bring much-needed warmth and energy to the place.

For the kidneys, hold your two hands over the small of your back. You may also want to book a couple of acupuncture appointments to help to unblock the area and bring energy back to the weakened organ.

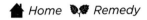

Ancient Chinese body talk: The meridian clock

The Chinese have understood the workings of the body for thousands of years. Until fairly recently, when technology and the latest modern scans finally 'proved' the existence of the invisible energy network of meridians and acupuncture points, Western medicine gave little credence to the concept of energy flow, nor to the physical problems that could arise when its flow was blocked. Traditional Chinese Medicine (TCM), however, is now accepted in the mainstream and acupuncture is widely available.

MERIDIAN CLOCK TEST

🏠 *Home*

TCM links different two-hour periods throughout the day and night to different organs of the body, and any repeat disturbance at a set time is said to be an indicator that a specific organ is weak. If you wake up at the same odd time every night, or early in the morning, you may have a problem. If you are waking at 2 a.m. every night, for example, it suggests that your liver is not working properly, and regularly waking at 4 a.m. indicates that your lungs are struggling. Consult a TCM practitioner for a specifically tailored herbal tonic, or a course of acupuncture, which will rebalance your energy system and boost whichever organs need help.

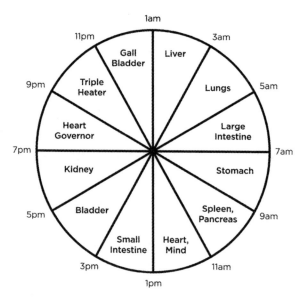

The meridian clock

TOP TIP

If you would like to find out whether any of your major glands or organs are not working properly, it is worth a visit to a kinesiologist or a NAET (Nambudripad's Allergy Elimination Technique) practitioner. These therapies monitor subtle muscle responses in the body, checking the energy flow in all your organs and systems, and identifying and clearing any blockages that might be preventing them functioning as well as they should.

Acid/alkaline balance

Keeping your body (measured through urine or saliva readings) as alkaline as possible is vital for your health, as many of its everyday processes produce acid and problems with any of your organs can create an overload of additional acid. Not to mention that many foods (e.g. fizzy drinks, processed foods, sugar, gluten, dairy and meat) also turn into acid and add to the burden. Moulds, bacteria, viruses and cancer cells in particular thrive in an acid environment[1] and struggle in an alkaline one, so becoming overly acid can allow disease to flourish. Keeping an eye on your pH balance is an effective way of avoiding that problem.

Your blood pH *always* stays the same at 7.365, so it's the pH of your saliva and urine that fluctuates and changes according to how you eat, drink and think. These are the pH levels that you can measure and will give you a picture of the health of your body tissues.

Simply put, your pH level measures how acid or alkaline you are. A pH of 0 is totally acid, 7 is neutral and at the other end of the scale a pH of 14 is totally alkaline. Ideally, your urine and saliva pH should be around 7.2–7.4. What you put in your mouth can alter the balance rapidly, so food is one of the most potent tools for boosting your health and balancing your alkalinity. Too alkaline a state, however, can also cause health problems, so work on a 70/30-alkaline/acid-food ratio and you will stay healthy.

In a nutshell, the acid-alkaline hypothesis states that acid-forming foods are bad for you and alkaline-forming foods are good.[2] This is because acid-forming foods are thought to raise your acid levels, affecting your bones and triggering poor health. Too much acid in your diet is also likely to be causing inflammation in the body. High stress levels also reduce your pH and make you more acidic. Feeling continually exhausted and craving sugar? Muscle or joint pains? Acidity is associated with tiredness and it can decrease your ability to absorb nutrients.

The problem can be easily reversed by a change in eating habits. To redress the balance, add more alkaline-forming 'healthy' foods – such as plenty of fresh fruits, vegetables and wholegrains – into your diet instead. You will become healthier and better protected against disease in the process.[3] As an added bonus, weight loss is a happy side-effect of balancing your pH.[4] Look online for charts with precise pH readings of specific foods and eat to adjust your balance.

Testing your saliva and urine is a simple way of getting a snapshot of your current physical health, and pH strips are inexpensive, easy to use and available on the Internet. The results will help you to assess the impact of what you are eating and work out if you need to change your diet. Urine should be more acidic and saliva alkaline, but the further apart your readings (i.e. very alkaline saliva and very acid urine), the greater your digestive problems are likely to be.

SALIVA PH STRIP TEST

🏠 *Home*

As soon as you wake up, test your saliva. Note the colour change on the strip and record the pH number. Do the test before you brush your teeth, drink anything, smoke or eat. An optimum saliva pH is 7. Digestive enzymes only get released efficiently when your levels are 6.5-7.

URINE PH STRIP TEST

🏠 *Home*

Urine is more acidic first thing in the morning, so it is best to take two readings in the day and average them out. Take readings a couple of times in the week over a few weeks to get a balanced overall picture.

Start by testing your first urine of the morning. This is urine that has been stored in your bladder during the night that is ready to be passed as soon as you get up. Simply hold a pH paper in your urine flow for a few moments and note the colour change to find the pH number.

The first urine should ideally have a pH of 6.8-7.2. Lower than 6.8 indicates there's a problem, but if your first urine pH is higher than 7.2, your alkaline buffers are sufficient to neutralize the acidic foods and drinks you ingested the day before.

Then test your second morning urine, before eating any food. This number will be the pH of your second wee of the day, after you have eliminated the acid load from the day before. The acids should be gone and ideally your urine pH should be 7.2 or higher. If your pH is lower than 6.8 then you are in a state of latent tissue acidosis, an indicator that you are deficient in alkaline buffers such as bicarbonate, sodium, potassium, magnesium and calcium. The lower pH is also suggestive of a diet that may indicate an overload of acids from too much protein, including nitric, sulphuric, phosphoric and uric acids. Cut the proportion of animal protein in your diet immediately, and increase the amount of green foods and healthy polyunsaturated fats.

Your urine pH should always be 7.2–8.4 right after meals and 6.5–7.2 a couple of hours after meals.

Understanding your results

Your pH level will tell you how acid or alkaline your body is.

The acid/alkaline scale runs from 0–14. Lower numbers, from 0–7 are considered acid and 7–14 more alkaline.

Different parts of the body have different healthy pH levels:

- Urine: 6.5–8

- Stomach: 1.5–2

- Digestive tract: 1.5–7.4

- Saliva 6.5–7

- Skin, which needs to be slightly acidic to keep off bacteria: 5.5

- Blood has the narrowest range of all at 7.35–7.45. The optimal pH of your blood is 7.365 and your body will do whatever it needs to keep it at that level, even depleting your bones and minerals in the process if needed.

Action plan

➔ **Drink apple cider vinegar:** If your pH is too acid, a daily drink of two tablespoons of raw, organic apple cider vinegar in hot water first thing in the morning will help to alkalize your body. It is antiviral, antifungal and antibacterial, and supports the immune system. It's also an acquired taste, but you quickly get fond of it.

➔ **Add in alkaline foods:** Including more alkaline foods will rapidly change your readings. Visit alkaline-diet-health-tips.com/alkaline-foods/alkaline-food-list for a comprehensive list of alkaline and acid foods.

➔ **Drink more:** Alkalizing water will help your body flush out.

➔ **Supplement:** Freeze-dried green power powders – *Chlorella*, algae or spirulina; barley or alfalfa grasses – will alkalize your body and increase your energy levels.

➔ **Drink green juice:** Drinking one green juice a day will alkalize your body and boost your immune system.

➔ **Reduce your stress levels:** Continual stress, whether it's physical, mental or emotional, raises your cortisol levels and triggers inflammation.[5] Psychological stress in particular distorts the body's anti-inflammatory reactions, and is linked to a build-up of free radicals and acidity, and serious health conditions such as depression, heart disease and cancer. Negative thoughts and feelings, and unresolved traumatic events, can literally make you sick. (See also Chapter 22.)

➔ **Breathe:** It takes between one and three minutes of deep breathing to change your pH and lower your acidity. Try Power Breathing: Inhale for two seconds, hold your breath for eight seconds and then exhale for four seconds. Repeat

10 times. Or meditate daily – even 10 minutes makes a difference (see Chapter 22, page 213).

Inflammation analysis

Inflammation is the secret trigger behind most disease;[5] it literally means that your body has an out-of-control fire raging somewhere inside you and indicates that there is severe irritation in the tissues and cells of the body.

Inflammation is the body's reaction to what it regards as a threat. It's an attempt to fight any invaders and a mechanism for triggering healing. Inflammation kicks in whenever you have a virus, unfriendly bacteria or wound, and in many ways and most instances, is a helpful, necessary process.

However, when your health is generally out of kilter, it can also become a chronic issue. When inflammation takes hold, it is usually a sign of the beginnings of health problems.

MIRROR TEST

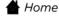 *Home*

Notice the following carefully when you look at yourself in the mirror: Is your face or body slightly swollen? Do you feel a bit puffy? Have you moved up a size in your clothes lately? It may not be weight gain but your body flagging something else is going on instead.

You might also want to take a photograph of your face today. After a two-week elimination diet, which involves excluding certain foods to test for food intolerances and sensitivities, take another. Note any differences.

CRP DIPSTICK TEST

🏠 *Home*

A CRP dipstick test from ultimed.org will give you accurate readings of your C-reactive protein levels and indicate how much inflammation your body is fighting.

BLOOD TEST

✚ *Doctor*

If you want further confirmation, double-check with your doctor and ask for a blood test. Your medical practitioner will be able to test for inflammatory markers in the blood through an ESR (erythrocyte sedimentation rate) test, during which the rate at which red blood cells fall to the bottom of the test tube is measured, or through a CRP test, which detects elevated protein levels in the blood, another indication of inflammation. Testing for 'inflammatory markers' in the blood is used in the diagnosis of a range of conditions from arthritis to Crohn's disease.[6]

Understanding your results

In your blood test, look for the results for fibrinogen, which measures inflammation in the tissues. The usual reference is a wide one, 100–500, but a healthy measurement should be 200–300. Another measure for inflammation is hs C-reactive protein (high-sensitivity C-reactive protein). The usual reference range is under 5, but a healthy marker should be under 1. If it is over 10, it usually means you have an infection rather than a systemic inflammation. Never test this one when you have a cold.

Action plan

→ **Change your diet:** Yet again, food is the key. Take out the foods that trigger inflammation, so avoid eating too much sugar, white flour products (i.e. biscuits, cakes), short-grain white rice, potatoes and processed cereals. Avoid MSG (monosodium glutamate), gluten and casein – in wheat, rye and whey products, and also aspartame and alcohol.

→ **Avoid bad fats:** Avoid saturated fats found in dairy products, meats and processed foods, as well as trans-fats in processed and fried foods. Avoid corn oil, vegetable oil, butter substitutes, shop-bought salad dressings and mayonnaise.

→ **Try a spice:** Turmeric (and curcumin, its potent anti-inflammatory extract) is reported to fight inflammation,[7] and can also help relieve rheumatoid arthritis and fibromyalgia symptoms such as stiffness in the morning, reducing swelling in the joints.[8] Take 1,200mg a day of curcumin, preferably in 300mg doses three times a day. Results show after two weeks of supplementation. You can incorporate turmeric into your daily diet by drinking Pukka Tea's 'Turmeric Gold'. Just one cup provides the same level of antioxidants as a bowl of blueberries. The compounds in the tea have been found to have anti-inflammatory, antidepressant and pain-relieving properties.

TOP TIP

To test for heavy metals, Lyme disease, gluten intolerance, candida, drug allergies and thiomersal, all triggers of inflammation in the body, visit melisa.org for an online test.

Test your sex hormones

Hormone imbalances can cause disruption throughout the body. Aside from low libido, a lack of testosterone in men and women can also increase weight gain, fatigue, high cholesterol, diabetes and depression.[9] High levels of testosterone in women play a part in the development of polycystic ovarian syndrome (PCOS).[10] Too little oestrogen causes brain fog and sleep difficulties, as well as low libido and exhaustion.[11] Too much, however, can cause weight gain, depression and tiredness.[12]

SALIVA TEST

🏠 *Home*

As we get older, hormone levels reduce and this can be behind many health issues. While blood hormone tests show which hormones are circulating in the bloodstream, saliva hormone tests give a more accurate picture of the quantity of hormones available to the body at a cellular level, the hormones that are actually being used by the body.

Saliva tests are simple, non-invasive and can be done at home. Together with a blood test, these two test results will give you a complete picture of your hormone health. Saliva tests can be bought from specialist labs on the Internet or via a qualified nutritionist, who can also talk you through the results and recommend the best course of treatment.

BLOOD TEST

✚ *Doctor*

Blood tests for hormones should be available through your doctor, and will show your levels of oestrogen, progesterone, DHEA (dehydroepiandrosterone) and testosterone, as well as your progesterone and estradiol ratio. Once you know where you are out of kilter, your doctor can advise the best course of treatment.

Menopause

Menopause is rarely talked about until you are actually in it, which is normally after the age of 50. No one really seems to know what to do about it, other than endure the hot flushes (also known as flashes), sweating, bloating, mind fog, low libido and weight gain, sometimes for years at a time, and pray for it to pass.

There are several ways that the female body deals with getting rid of toxins – through the bowels, the liver, the kidneys and, the one that differs from their male counterparts, via their periods. When the latter finally stops at menopause, a major part of the normal detox process is thrown off and unbalanced, so your body has to find other ways to get rid of what it needs to.

Your GP may offer you HRT (hormone replacement therapy) to balance whatever hormones are out. These artificial hormones do relieve many of the symptoms that often accompany menopause, but can also cause side-effects that include headaches, breast tenderness and bloating. More serious problems include increased chances of blood clots, hormone-related cancers, heart disease and stroke. Please inform yourself about the pros and cons of taking HRT first. There are vociferous 'for' and 'against' camps. There is no scientific evidence that supports continuing with the treatment after the age of 60.

If you, for whatever reason, go into menopause early (and around 8 per cent of women will) or your periods stop prematurely (POI – primary ovarian insufficiency), perhaps because you have had chemotherapy or radiotherapy or had a full hysterectomy, you will have a higher risk of developing osteoporosis due to reduced oestrogen levels. Your doctor will recommend you take HRT to support your hormones until you reach the age when you would normally have become menopausal, which is around your early 50s.

Action plan

→ **Strengthen your organs:** How well your kidneys and liver function is a major factor in how easily you get through menopause, so consider doing a kidney and a liver cleanse, which may help relieve the intensity of your symptoms (see Chapter 7, page 84).

→ **Regulate hormones:** Coffee, alcohol, cigarettes and spicy foods can all aggravate menopause symptoms and so are best avoided.

➜ **Keep cool:** Keep your room cold at night and invest in a fan. A cold temperature keeps your body temperature better in check.

➜ **Use CBT (cognitive behavioural therapy):** CBT can help reduce the anxiety and helplessness so often associated with menopause. CBT helps you change the messaging in your mind and researchers found that four sessions were enough to reduce the number and severity of hot flushes significantly.

➜ **Up your exercise:** Exercise really does make a difference. Endorphins released during exercise ease anxiety and depression and those low moods frequently associated with menopause.

➜ **Experiment with essential oils:** Clary sage oil is frequently flagged as the most effective of the essential oils for balancing hormones. It reduces anxiety and lessens hot flushes. Roman chamomile oil reduces stress, peppermint oil can help cool the body from hot flushes, and thyme oil and basil oil help to balance hormones naturally. Try rubbing basil oil across the back of your neck to help cool you down. A research study on citrus oil in 2014 found that postmenopausal women who inhaled it regularly experienced fewer physical symptoms and an increase in sexual desire. Citrus also has anti-inflammatory properties, and can help ease the joint aches and pains associated with menopause.[13]

➜ **Try herbal medicine:** Consult a medical herbalist or naturopath for a personalized prescription tailored to your specific symptoms. Herbs and natural plant medicine shown to help with menopausal symptoms include red clover, maca, evening primrose oil, liquorice root, wild yams, red raspberry leaves and sarsaparilla. Chasteberry, or agnus castus, has been clinically proven to regulate hormones and lessen hot flushes. Black cohosh stops night sweats and hot flushes and improves sleep. Proper dosages and combinations are important here, so please don't just self-prescribe.

→ **Up your vitamin D levels:** Research shows that the lower your vitamin D levels, the more likely you are to suffer from menopausal symptoms.[14] Check with your doctor and get a blood test to identify your levels. And be guided by his or her advice, because overly high levels can cause as many problems as deficiency. Many people are deficient or low in vitamin D, so supplement and get your levels up (see the Appendix).

→ **Lose weight if you can:** You may find you put on additional pounds and struggle to lose them with all the hormonal fluctuations. Your body will try to hold on to as much oestrogen-producing fat as possible as your customary oestrogen levels wane. Testosterone levels drop during menopause too, which slows down your metabolic rate. Eating the same amount as usual will increase your weight, so cut your processed food consumption. If you are having a particularly bad time with your menopause, the stress of the situation will raise your cortisol levels too, and increase fat around your stomach. (See also Chapters 2 and 7.)

TOP TIP

A small, inexpensive magnet has been developed that seems to reduce substantially or stop menopausal symptoms. The LadyCare is said to work for more than

80 per cent of the women who have tried it. It is also effective at combating the muscle aches, hot flushes and other side-effects of chemotherapy (ladycare-uk.com).

Pyroluria

Pyroluria is a little-known imbalance in the production of a group of chemicals called kryptopyrroles, which causes the body continually to dump both B6 and zinc into the urine. B6 is essential for brain and nervous system health, whilst zinc affects mood, and zinc deficiency causes anxiety and depression. There is also a well-established link between anorexia and lack of zinc.[15] If nothing else seems to have made much of a difference, it's well worth taking this test.

If you have pyroluria, you will pass more urine than usual – often more than 3 litres (6 pints) a day, and usually a lot in one go rather than little and often. The higher your level of stress, the faster the body gets rid of the B6 and zinc, and the more severe the symptoms.

On average, 11 per cent of us suffer from pyroluria and it is abnormally high in people with mental health problems: 40 per cent of alcoholics have pyroluria, 30 per cent of schizophrenics and 40 per cent of people with psychiatric issues.[16]

PYROLURIA CHECKLIST

 Home

Answer the following questions yes or no:

1. Did you sunburn easily when you were young? Do you have the palest skin and hair in your family?

2. Do you have thin hair, eyebrows and eyelashes or prematurely grey hair?

3. Do you have poor dream recall or nightmares?

4. Are you becoming more of a loner as you age? Do you avoid stressful situations?

5. Have you been anxious, fearful or felt a lot of inner tension since childhood, but mostly repress these feelings?

6. Is it hard to recall past events and people in your life?

7. Do you have bouts of depression and/or nervous exhaustion?

8. Do you have cluster headaches?

9. Are your eyes sensitive to sunlight?

10. Do you belong to all-female family or have lookalike sisters?

11. Do you get frequent colds or infections, or unexplained chills or fevers?

12. Do you dislike eating protein? Have you ever been a vegetarian?

13. Did you reach puberty later than normal?

14. Are there white flecks on your fingernails, or do you have opaque white or thin nails? Are you a nail-biter?

15. Are you prone to acne, eczema or psoriasis?

16. Are you anaemic?

17. Do you have cold hands/feet?

18. Do you have a tendency to be constipated in the mornings?

19. Do you have tingling sensations or muscle spasms in your legs/arms?

20. Do you prefer the company of one or two close friends, rather than large gatherings?

21. Do you have stretch marks?

22. Do your knees crack or ache?

23. Have you noticed that your breath has a sweet or fruity odour when you're stressed?

24. Do you have, or did you have before braces, crowded upper front teeth?

25. Do you prefer not to eat breakfast or experience mild nausea in the morning?

26. Does your face sometimes look swollen when under stress?

27. Do you have a poor appetite, or poor sense of smell or taste?

28. Do you have any upper abdominal or spleen pain? As a child, did you get a stitch when you ran or exercised?

29. Do you tend to focus internally on yourself, rather than the outside world?

30. Do you regularly experience fatigue?

31. Do you feel uncomfortable with strangers?

32. Do tranquillizers, alcohol or other drugs produce an unusually strong response in you?

33. Do you dislike being seated in the middle of a room, rather than at the sides?

34. Are you easily upset by criticism?

35. Do changes in your routine provoke stress?

36. Do you tend to be dependent on one person?

Understanding your results

Circulating levels of pyroles may be slightly elevated or profoundly abnormal. In all cases, these levels rise even more when under stress, so if you are B6 and zinc deficient, you will easily identify with many of the aforementioned questions. If you score 15 or more, it may well be worth being tested for pyroluria.

Don't panic if you score high on the test. The problem is simple to sort. A pyroluria blood test is available (pyroluriatesting.com), and once you have a confirmed result, you can begin supplementation.

Action plan

→ **Use Bio-Recovery's pyroluria product:** Available from bio-recoveryinc.com, this supplement offers a specific combination formula for pyroluria, which includes B6, zinc, pyridoxal-5-phosphate, manganese, magnesium, niacinamide, pantothenic acid and vitamin C, and can relieve symptoms in three weeks. If you are diagnosed with pyroluria you will need to take the supplements for the rest of your life and whenever you are suffering from severe stress, up the dosage to stay balanced and healthy.

Vitamin D deficiency

Probably the most important test of all is for vitamin D, as every tissue and cell in your body has a receptor for it, which makes it a hormone – most confusing. But either way, you really, really need it. Low levels of vitamin D can trigger a wide range of health issues, including depression, inflammation, allergies, autoimmune symptoms, diabetes[17-19] and many cancers. Vitamin D helps regulate the absorption of calcium, phosphate and magnesium from the gut, and is essential for the development of strong bones. A Public Health England Government report, published in 2007, showed that nearly three quarters of the population are low in vitamin D.[20] Supplementing by taking vitamin D3 protects against lung, breast, prostate, ovarian and colon cancer.

Vitamin D is made in the skin and then moves through your blood to the liver and the kidneys, and helps the bones absorb calcium, keeping them strong. Deficiency is linked to osteoporosis and bone weakness,[21] heart problems,[22] depression,[23] back pain, insulin resistance and macular degeneration, as well as cancer,[24] rheumatoid arthritis, IBS, MS and diabetes.[24] Low levels are associated with weight gain.[25]

If you have darker skin you may need as much as 10 times more sun exposure to produce the same amount of vitamin D as a person with paler skin. And if you're over 55 it is harder for your skin to produce vitamin D through sun exposure.

The main source of vitamin D is sunlight, but in the northern hemisphere, from October to March, the angle of the sun is too low for the UVB rays to penetrate your skin and trigger production. During this time, we have to rely on our own stores, vitamin D found in some foods or vitamin D3 supplements.[26]

VITAMIN D3 TEST

🏠 *Home*

Vitamindtest.org.uk offers an inexpensive D3 test for home use.

BLOOD TEST

✚ *Doctor*

Ask your doctor to give you a blood test for vitamin D – 25 OH-VIT D (VitD2+D3). There are two types of vitamin D – D2 and D3 (always supplement with D3), and this test establishes the amount you have available of each. Over half of us are deficient, so it is important to supplement daily, especially during the winter.

Understanding your results

- Below 10ng/ml – severe deficiency
- 10–19ng/ml – deficiency
- 20–29ng/ml – insufficiency
- 30–50ng/ml – optimal
- 51–99ng/ml – minor excess
- Over 100ng/ml – excessive

To reach an optimal level of 50ng/ml, you'll need to take 2,000IU daily (and 100IU of additional D3 for each 1ng/ml you want to raise it). In one research study, 3,320IU daily was found to reduce triglycerides by 13.5 per cent. Weight loss and better HDL cholesterol levels were additional side-effects. Breastfeeding mothers are now recommended to take 400IU daily of vitamin D in order to boost their baby's levels, because breast milk itself contains less than 50IU's per quart.

Action plan

➜ **Supplement daily:** If you are low in vitamin D, supplement with vitamin D3 combined with K2, and take vitamin A too, so that the body can synthesize vitamin D properly. Spray-type supplements get vitamin D into your body faster than in pill or capsule form.

➜ **Take vitamin D with a meal:** The fats in the food help the body absorb it 50 per cent better.[27]

> *TOP TIP*
>
> *Different supplements work differently for different people, which means your body might not be absorbing vitamin D, despite supplementing. Make sure you check your vitamin D levels regularly to check your numbers are increasing. If they aren't, try another brand. Test at different times of year and keep track of your levels.*

➜ **Get outside:** The sun is the best source of vitamin D. Aim for at least 20 minutes a day outdoors and try to keep your arms, legs or face exposed. The best time for light metabolism for the body is before 9 a.m. or two hours before sunset. This only works April–October in the northern hemisphere. During winter, your levels will be lower and you must supplement. Or go on regular holidays somewhere sunny.

→ **Eat vitamin D boosting foods:** The best source of vitamin D is oily fish, like salmon, sardines, mackerel and tuna. Cheese and egg yolks are good, as are mushrooms and raw (unpasteurized) milk, plus any vitamin D fortified foods (usually cereals, orange juice and dairy products).

Histamine

An overload of copper can lead to imbalances in histamine, a chemical that is released as part of the body's allergic response and stimulates the response of the neurotransmitters that govern mood within the brain. This can have an impact on everything from libido to energy.[28]

When balanced, histamine creates a feeling of emotional stability in the brain. It works in the hypothalamus to stimulate the release of serotonin, dopamine and norepinephrine, which are neurotransmitters responsible for mood balance, concentration and alertness. Too little histamine, however, raises dopamine levels, and can trigger a wide range of psychological and physical symptoms.

It is 100 per cent possible to balance histamine through diet, but first you'll need to identify and then rebalance the body's copper levels, as excess copper decreases histamine levels in the brain. A blood test that measures histamine will determine whether or not you have an issue, and a hair mineral analysis test, available either online or from a nutritionist, can analyse the levels of copper in your body. (See Chapter 24, page 233.)

Action plan

→ **Balance histamine:** Ask your doctor for advice to balance histamine levels and reduce copper levels. Reduce protein and up your consumption of fruit and vegetables.

→ **Supplement:** Bio-recoveryinc.com offers a formula package for low histamine. If you have high histamine levels, the amino acid methionine will lower your numbers when taken 500mg four times daily. Calcium and magnesium supplements are also recommended. High histamine influences mood, sleep, appetite and thought processes, and the biochemical imbalance in a high-histamine person can lead to depression, perfectionism and OCD (obsessive compulsive disorder).[29]

Part II

Boosting Health – Body and Mind

'It is health that is real wealth and not pieces of gold and silver.'

MAHATMA GANDHI

Chapter 19

Food Fundamentals

*'The food you eat can be either the safest
and most powerful form of medicine
or the slowest form of poison.'*

ANN WIGMORE

Food promotes wellbeing and provides us with the energy we need to thrive. In fact, did you know that the food you eat has an almost immediate effect on your body and your biochemistry changes within a few minutes of eating a meal? You become what you eat – literally.

However, the advice on what we should and shouldn't eat is often confusing and seems to change regularly. Take butter, for example. One moment it's labelled as bad and margarine or 'spreads' as good or better, and the next margarine is toxic and butter is the best option. Or eggs: cholesterol baddies or superfood? Sometimes it's hard to trust information from the food industry or the scientists it funds and many people also (wisely) feel equally sceptical when it comes to government advice.

But the simple truth is that you probably already know what constitutes a healthy diet: nourishing, whole foods that improve wellbeing. We know that the body thrives on fruits and vegetables, the healthy fats and proteins found in foods like avocados, nuts and oily fish; and that processed or fast food, sugars, saturated fats, alcohol and caffeine don't serve us... and in this chapter, we'll explore how you can restore health through diet.

Eating dos and don'ts

Now you've been through the tests in Part I, you're probably aware of which organs and systems need more support. But the first place to start, whatever your health issue, is by giving your body a break from any eating habits that may be harming your wellbeing. Secondly, you need to add in healthier foods to ensure that you're eating a wide and balanced diet. You don't have to make these changes overnight, just start shifting away from the bad stuff and towards more of the good stuff, and the following rules are probably the most beneficial in helping you choose what to eat:

Do eat

Organic: Organic produce may be more expensive, but it has more nutrients and fewer chemicals. It's particularly important to opt for organic produce when you eat the peel.

Fresh: Exposure to light and air destroys nutrients in foods in the space of a few days, so keep your eye on best-before dates and regularly replenish your stocks.

A balanced diet: Eat a wide range of foods, but focus on wholegrains, nuts and seeds, large quantities of fresh vegetables, and some fruit, pulses and plenty of water.

Raw: Aim for 50:50, because uncooked food is full of enzymes and releases huge amounts of energy, so opt for salads or juices and smoothies whenever possible. The pancreas, for example, can repair itself entirely after six weeks on a restricted raw, plant-based diet.[1]

Cooking food in temperatures over 48°C (118°F) destroys 100 per cent of the enzymes, and 50 per cent of its minerals and vitamins. Vanderbilt University found that cooked foods contained 60–70 per cent of the iron calcium, copper, magnesium, manganese, phosphorus, potassium, sodium and zinc found in uncooked foods,[2-3] while boiled, soaked, fried or stewed vegetables lost the most minerals. Thiamine, folic acid and vitamins B6 and C are especially affected by cooking, and steamed foods retain the most nutrients.

Good oils: Opt for cold-pressed organic oils. If you heat your oils, cook with coconut oil, rapeseed oil, butter or ghee. Drizzle cold-pressed olive oil or avocado oil onto cold or cooked dishes and salads. Good fats (e.g. coconut, olive, sesame, avocado and flaxseed oil, and cod liver and fish oils) help the brain to work properly, and balance your mood and hormones.

Less meat: Choose lean cuts of grass-fed and organic meats whenever possible. Hormones, antibiotics, pesticides and other chemicals are an integral part of production nowadays, and meat is increasingly being linked to the development of disease. Processed meat – e.g. cured, salted, smoked or preserved meats such as bacon, sausages, ham, salami and pepperoni – has been classified by the International Agency for Research on Cancer (IARC) as a 'definite' cause of cancer, based on the results of more than 800 studies.[4] Red meat – beef, lamb and pork – is considered a 'probable' cause.[5] Fresh chicken, turkey or fish do not appear to increase cancer risks.

A rainbow: Try to include as many colours as possible in your choice of fruit and vegetables, as each colour contains different nutrients for health.

Smaller portions: Your stomach is only the size of your fist, so eat less and more often. Eat slowly, put your knife and fork down between mouthfuls, eat mindfully and chew each morsel 20 times before swallowing – it releases saliva that helps digest the food well.

Carefully stored food: Heat changes the chemical structure of fats, proteins and vitamins in foods, reducing their nutritional content, and affecting both the flavour and often the smell. Light and exposure to oxygen also affects vitamin C levels, so it's vital to make sure your food is stored properly. Although scientific debate still rages about the nutritional impact of microwaving food, it's best to avoid it if you can because the jury is still out as regards its safety.

> *TOP TIP*
>
> *The ETE plate (eteplate.com) can help you control portion size, as it is divided into sections to ensure you eat the optimal amount of protein, carbohydrate and vegetables in each meal.*

Avoid

Anything that didn't exist 500 years ago: In other words, highly processed, refined or fast foods.

Chemicals, additives, etc.: If you can't understand the names of the ingredients on the label or pack, don't eat it.

GMO: Any genetically modified (GMO) foods, as science has yet to prove their safety.[6]

Anything that doesn't seem to agree with you: If a food leaves you feeling bloated, fatigued or generally unwell, don't eat it.

'Bad' fats (including saturated fats, i.e. animal and dairy produce, and trans-fats, which are in many processed foods): Don't eat margarine or any other olive oil/butter margarine substitutes or spreads. Although most no longer contain trans-fats, they often contain palm oil (a serious threat to cardiovascular health and the environment), are highly processed and bad news for health.[7] A better option is to eat organic butter in moderation, as it contains vitamins A, D, K and E, antioxidants, selenium and iodine. Raw butter has even more health compounds.

Eating fruit at the end of a meal: Fruit digests fast, so it needs to be eaten first, otherwise it gets trapped behind slower foods and ferments in the stomach.

Drinking with your meal: We all do it – the table setting encourages it with that nice tumbler full of water sitting in front of you just waiting to be drunk. Lay the table without glasses for a few days. Eat without drinking and see if you notice the difference. Try to drink your glass of water or wine 20 minutes before you sit down to eat instead. Liquid dilutes your digestive juices, so once again, the foods you have eaten won't get broken down properly and your stomach will suffer.

> ## TOP TIP
>
> *If you suffer with digestive problems, bloating and gas, then try adding a pinch of hing or asafoetida powder to your food. You can usually buy it in Indian food stores, but beware, it's not called 'Devil's Dung' for nothing! But worth the stench – it really works.*

Toxins: When choosing tinned food, opt for varieties labelled 'BPA free'. Many tinned foods are contaminated with bisphenol A, a toxic chemical that has been shown to cause reproductive abnormalities, brain damage, breast and prostate cancer, diabetes, heart disease and other serious health problems. Tomatoes are particularly high in acid, which causes even more BPA to leach into the food. A better option is to choose food sold in glass jars. I know it's not always easy, but it's best to avoid plastic packaging too. And if you have to buy it, check the number on the bottom of the product, which is usually found inside a recycling symbol. The numbers range from 1 to 7 and identify the type of plastic used: 2, 4 and 5 are the safer choices, while 3, 6 and 7 are the particularly toxic combinations.

Vegetable oils, such as sunflower oil, corn oil and soybean oil: Many are highly processed and heat-treated, causing chemical changes that can damage your health. When the oil is heated and mixed with oxygen, it goes rancid. Too much omega-6 (the type of fat found in these oils) is associated with a range of health problems and vegetable oil that's reheated (such as deep-fat fryer oil) is loaded with trans-fats.

Non-organic fruits and vegetables: Opt for organic apples, peaches, celery, potatoes, spinach, tomatoes, nectarines, cucumbers, pears, grapes, strawberries and peppers because of the 48 different foods tested by the EWG (Environmental Working Group)[8] these had the highest pesticide load. Even after washing they still contain 67 per cent of these nasties.

Too much salt: Whether it's table salt, rock salt, sea salt or a flavoured salt like garlic or celery, salt is salt and eating too much has negative health consequences. Salt has high sodium chloride levels, which increases your blood pressure and thus your chance of strokes and heart problems.[9] A little salt in your diet is a good thing, but choose wisely.

Table salt is a highly processed product and so best avoided. It contains many manufactured chemicals which are toxic to the human body, including fluoride, synthetic iodide, aluminium derivatives and anti-caking agents.[10] A better option is Himalayan or Celtic salt, as these have slightly higher levels of calcium, potassium, magnesium and iron.[11] The pinkish Himalayan sea salt still contains 85 per cent sodium chloride, but it also contains 84 trace minerals, with no heavy metals or industrial toxins. A small amount of Himalayan salt is said to regulate blood pressure, assist the brain to work and carry nutrients to the cells; though there are few scientific studies available to back this up. In addition, research shows that Himalayan salt effectively 're-mineralized' the bodies of participants in a 2007 trial, also stabilizing pH and oxidative stress numbers. A 2001 Austrian study found significant changes in sleep, energy and weight loss, and noticeable hair and nail growth.[12]

Processed soya products: The jury is still out on the health benefits of soya, but the argument seems to be linked to whether it is processed or organic and properly fermented. Long promoted as a healthy alternative to dairy, unfermented soya products have been linked with malnutrition, thyroid problems, brain dysfunction and digestive issues in hundreds of studies.[13-14] In the USA, 95 per cent of soya beans are genetically engineered and these can upset female hormone balance, raising oestrogen levels and affecting fertility. The only soya with health benefits is organic soya found in fermented products such as miso, tempeh and certain soy sauces, tofu and soymilk. The fermentation creates the probiotics, the 'good' bacteria, such as *Lactobacillus* (see also Chapter 4, page 50).

Artificial sweeteners: Did you know that saccharin and aspartame can cause greater weight gain than sugar?[15] Even though they only contain a few or zero calories, artificial sweeteners stimulate appetite and increase carbohydrate cravings. Aspartame, found in many diet fizzy drinks, has also been shown to alter the microbiome of the gut, and is associated with high blood pressure, depression and migraine headaches, as well as increasing your risk of developing Type 2 diabetes by 67 per cent.[16-17] A better option is to swap the sugar in your bowl for stevia, a natural plant product that has no calories and has been shown to lower blood pressure.[18]

Nutrient thieves: Alcohol, caffeine, nicotine, sugar, aspartame and salt all destroy nutrients and stop your body from properly absorbing, using and digesting them. Coffee and tea deplete vitamin B complex and vitamin C, and reduce iron absorption. Smoking reduces vitamin E levels by up to 45 per cent and lowers vitamin A levels. Excess alcohol intake also affects vitamin A and fat metabolism.

TOP TIPS

- *If you suffer from disturbed sleep, avoiding drinking alcohol and caffeine in the evening. Both are stimulants and stay in your system for several hours, triggering dehydration and causing you to wake up in the night with a dry mouth and headache. Drink a glass or two of water before you sleep to dilute their effect. Also avoid eating heavy meals late at night. Before bed, try camomile or valerian[19] tea – nature's alternative sleeping pill.*

- *Cut out the sugar: Sugar is the big no-no because not only is it addictive and often genetically modified to boot, but it also causes your blood sugar levels to spike and crash – and long term that can deliver you into the jaws of diabetes with all of its associated health issues. All carbohydrates turn into sugar, whether it's the piece of white toast you have for breakfast or the bowl of pasta for lunch. It's just a question of the amount of time it takes to give you that short-lived high. And did you know that a glass of orange juice has the same amount of sugar as a can of cola?*

If in doubt about what to eat, remember the following acronyms:

Eat Less **CRAP**

C – carbonated drinks

R – refined sugar

A – artificial sweeteners and colours

P – Processed foods

Eat more **FOOD**

F – Fruits and vegetables

O – Organic meat

O – Omega-3 oils

D – Drink more water

Superfoods

Superfoods are plant medicines, packed full of vitamins, minerals and antioxidants that can turbocharge your wellbeing. Rapidly absorbed, they are antiviral, anti-inflammatory and repair the immune system, and most of them taste pretty good too. A couple of teaspoons in a daily smoothie will boost your energy levels. Try them out and find the ones that work for you.

Benefits of superfoods	
Acai	Brazilian berry. Reduces high blood pressure[20]
Astragalus	Anti-ageing, immune system booster – a 'bug' protector against flu and germs[21]
Ashwagandha	Ayurveda herb that helps with memory and sleep, calms and strengthens the nerves[22]
Bee pollen	A multivitamin in a single food – anti-inflammatory, antiallergic, helps circulation and heart, slows ageing[23]
Cacao	Boosts endorphins – must eat raw[24]
Chia	An energy-giving Mayan grain, high in protein and omega-3[25]
Cinnamon	Balances blood sugar, stabilizes sugar cravings and an anti-inflammatory[26]
Goji berries	'The key to eternal youth' according to the Tibetans and also good for eye health[27]
Green tea	Boosts metabolism, lowers cholesterol and calms yet energizes the brain[28]
Hemp	Brain and immune booster, repairs and builds muscle and an anti-inflammatory for joint pain[29]
Maca	Used by the Incas for energy and stress reduction, it is good for bones and menopause[30-31]
Olive leaf	Boosts immune system and a good anticold and antiflu remedy,[32-33] it also relieves candida, gout and arthritis[34]
Rhodiola	Siberian herb that regulates stress,[35] increases serotonin and is good for depression
Spirulina	A high-protein algae (65–70 per cent), it is a blood purifier, and improves cholesterol and arthritis[36]
Turmeric	Strengthens digestion, improves liver function and helps with joint pain[37]
Wheatgrass	Alkalizes body, and stimulates thyroid and metabolism[38]

Broad-spectrum supplements

Broad-spectrum products are 100 per cent natural wholefoods in a form that can be easily absorbed and used by your body – just like food itself.[39] Among others, barley grass, Chlorella, bee pollen, royal jelly and spirulina are all reputed to be potent healers, rebooting energy levels and upping immunity. Each one contains large amounts of vitamins, minerals, trace elements, amino acids, polysaccharides, essential fatty acids, nucleic acids, micronutrients, carbohydrates, sterols, fats, protein and fibre. All of these nutrients work together to create health benefits that cannot be achieved by the synthetic supplements.

> **TOP TIP**
>
> *Include some blue-green algae in your diet, as it reboots your cells and rebuilds the mitochondria that rule them. Only buy freeze-dried algae and take it first thing in the morning. Within three months you should be thinking and remembering better than before. Blue-green algae has been shown to help with Alzheimer's and brain injury, increase energy, vitality and stamina, as well as stress, depression and anxiety; and it boosts the immune system.[40]*

Nutritional supplements

Many conventional doctors and health advisers say that there should be no need to supplement if you eat a balanced diet. However, modern lifestyles and eating habits, as well as the paucity of nutrients in the soil due to modern farming practices and intensive pesticide use, mean that much of the food we eat is nutritionally depleted.[41] Within the alternative health community, there's a consensus that supplementing is a good idea, but the vast range of vitamins, minerals and herbs can feel confusing, so where should you start?

You'll find a list of some of the most important vitamins and minerals, with an explanation of what they do, in the Appendix (see page 253). Depending on your specific health issue, choose which ones might be right for you and supplement accordingly. It can be as bad to overdose on a supplement as to be low in it, so it's always best to know what you need by double-checking your requirements with a qualified naturopathic doctor or nutritionist. Complementary practitioners often offer full body scans on biofeedback machines that can tell you what minerals and vitamins you lack.[42]

TOP TIPS

- *For a detailed analysis of your mineral and vitamin needs, try Vitastiq, an inexpensive hand-held probe that connects to your smartphone and will give you an accurate reading of 30 essential vitamins and minerals (vitastiq.com).*

- *Some pharmaceutical pills, especially statins and steroids, alongside laxatives and antacids, have a negative effect too. Take supplements to top up your vitamin and mineral levels, but make sure you take them with water, rather than hot drinks that can destroy their contents.*

Action plan

→ **Don't go mad and buy the lot:** If you build a giant collection of pills and potions, you may feel overwhelmed by how many you need to consume each day – and they can be expensive too. Follow the dosage recommendations.

→ **Write a list of which supplements are good for your symptoms:** Just choose a few to start and finish one bottle before you start on the next. Be patient, as you'll need to take some supplements for a month or two before you begin to see an improvement.

➜ **Choose natural products:** Many supplements are synthetic, made to replicate the natural product, but with altered molecules that may mean that your body is not able to utilize them efficiently, so choose broad-spectrum supplements wherever possible (see page 183). Taking supplements in a liquid drop or liposomal form under your tongue is the fastest way of getting them into your body.

➜ **Take a break:** It's never a good idea to supplement for too long with the same products, so take a break for a while every few months or so. Fundamentally important supplements should be considered long-term health aids, but from time to time change the brand. And if you're not sure where to start, try the following plan:

~ Multivitamin

~ Multimineral

~ Combined omega-3 and -6 oil

~ Vitamin D3 and K2 in spray form

~ B-complex formula

~ Vitamin C separately

~ Zinc

~ Probiotics

~ Digestive and systemic enzymes

~ Then choose according to your health issue

TOP TIP

Some brands are reliable and do what they say on the packet – others do not. ConsumerLab.com is a website that tests a range of products for every vitamin, mineral and health supplement on the market for quality and efficacy. They grade the suppliers, so you can be safe in the knowledge that what you're putting in your body is the best available. There is an annual charge for the service, but the website does gives you access to literally thousands of up-to-date tests on a vast range of products.

When to take supplements

What supplements you need depends on your lifestyle and although taking them spread out throughout the day may be optimal, if you are likely to forget then it's probably best to swallow them all at once in the mornings at breakfast. If you have larger quantities of pills to take, buy some small plastic bags and take your daily quota with you to work to take whenever recommended. Always take supplements 15 minutes before or after a meal.

Understanding your appetite

Before we finish this chapter, I'd also like to share the importance of understanding how appetite can affect your eating habits, particularly if you're struggling with weight loss due to feeling hungry all the time.

Leptin and ghrelin are the two hormones responsible for regulating your appetite, and therefore your weight. By sending signals to the hypothalamus in the brain, leptin decreases hunger and ghrelin stimulates it.[43] If you feel hungry, you eat more. The more you eat, the more weight you gain. In a perfect world, the two should keep your eating habits and your weight in balance. All sorts of factors, however, can cause you to become resistant to one or the other or both. Weight gain seems to be the main one, which messes up your brain signals, triggering yet more weight gain and fat retention.

Leptin is mainly produced by your fat cells and is often called the master hormone because it controls body weight. Leptin regulates your appetite and metabolism. If leptin production is optimal it can aid weight loss, but if not it could make it harder to lose any excess weight.

If your diet contains too many carbohydrates and too much sugar, the sugar turns to fat and gets stored around your middle. The fatter you get, the higher your leptin levels rise, until eventually, as with insulin, your body becomes resistant. You receive hunger signals and eat more and more, and as you get fatter, your leptin levels get higher and higher. Your brain can't read the messages and it can't tell that you are overweight, increasing your chance of high blood pressure, stroke and heart disease. It becomes a vicious circle.

Ghrelin is produced in the stomach lining when it is empty and its function is to increase your appetite, sending hunger signals directly to the brain. Japanese scientists only discovered its existence in 1999 and there are currently no tests available to identify your levels. If you are constantly yo-yoing with your weight and put it straight back on after dieting, you may have found your answer.[44]

Ghrelin levels increase before meals and then decrease after them, for up to three hours. Lack of sleep can also increase ghrelin levels.[45] Eating disorders, such as anorexia and bulimia, trigger the release of higher levels of the hormone, to create hunger pangs and encourage eating.[46]

If you think grehlin or leptin may be a problem for you, the best way to reduce this weight gain is to change your diet, cutting down on carbohydrates and processed foods, and eating as many raw foods as possible.

Action plan

→ Eat every 4 hours.

→ Start your day with protein.

→ Eat more high-fibre foods.

→ Avoid fructose and MSG.

→ Eat more good fats; they trigger feelings of satiety that helps reduce cravings for empty carbs.

→ Take fish oil supplements; omega-3 fatty acids are linked to decreased hunger.

→ Reduce your stress levels. (See also Chapter 22.)

→ Get a good night's sleep, as lack of sleep increases ghrelin and decreases leptin. (See also Chapter 23.)

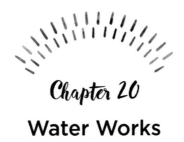

Chapter 20

Water Works

'Drinking water is like washing out your insides. The water will cleanse the system, fill you up, decrease your caloric load and improve the function of all your tissues.'

KEVIN R. STONE

M any medical practitioners and official bodies recommend drinking five glasses of water a day, but say that fruit juice or other drinks can count too. Others say eight glasses of water a day, and some recommendations go as high as 3 litres (6 pints) daily for men and 2.2 litres (4½ pints) for women. Within these guidelines, most experts agree that the exact amount varies from person to person.

You're likely to drink about 75,000 litres (almost 20,000 gallons) of water in your lifetime, but some people don't drink enough, or substitute coffee, tea and soft drinks, not realizing that these actually act as diuretics, triggering dehydration. Drinking water – pure water with nothing in it – is vital for health, as 80 per cent of your brain, 90 per cent of your blood and 96 per cent of your liver consists of water.[1] Water is involved in nearly every chemical reaction in your body; it regulates body temperature, carries nutrients to your cells and tissues, and carries toxins away and disposes of them. Water protects your organs and tissue, and helps with the digestion, absorption and elimination of food.

We lose water every day – through breathing, moving, sweating, exercising and urinating – and a simple way to tell whether or not you're drinking enough is to look at the colour of your urine; it should be pale yellow and odourless. If your urine is dark yellow, then you probably need to drink more water. And remember, hot weather increases water loss, as does fever or illness.

If the amount of water in your body is reduced by just 1 per cent, you'll feel thirsty, but 75 per cent of us are regularly dehydrated. We can live without food for about a month, but only three to seven days without water. And there are many other benefits to drinking enough, including:

- Drinking 2 litres (4¼ pints) of water a day can increase energy expenditure by about 96 calories per day.[2]

- If you drink cold water, the body has to use energy (calories) to heat it to body temperature. Room temperature water is less shocking to the gut.

- Drinking water about 30 minutes before meals can reduce the number of calories you eat. In one study, dieters who drank 500ml (1 pint) of water before meals lost 44 per cent more weight over a period of 12 weeks, compared to those who didn't, as metabolic rate increases by 30 per cent for up to 40 minutes.[3]

- Even mild dehydration can slow down your metabolism as much as 3 per cent, and increase feelings of anxiety and tiredness.[4]

- Dehydration can trigger anxiety and depression, chronic fatigue and attention deficit disorder (ADD).[5]

- It takes roughly three glasses of water to neutralize the caffeine in one cup of tea or coffee.

- Drinking about 2 litres (4¼ pints) water daily can help you stay hydrated, and cause headaches and back and joint pain to vanish.[6]

- Dehydration is a major cause of early afternoon tired time.

> **TOP TIP**
>
> *The Camelbak hydration calculator (camelbak.com) can help you to work out your ideal hydration level. Just tap in your gender, height, weight and age, and hey presto, get drinking.*

What's in your drinking water?

Tap water often contains small amounts of toxic chemicals, such as fluoride, arsenic, chlorine, metals, nitrates and other substances that have been shown to be the cause of health problems.[7-8] Drinking it, cooking with it or bathing in it – what is in the water, goes into your body.

Your drinking water travels through many kilometres of pipes to get to your tap and into your kettle or your water glass. As well as contamination from pipes, there are also bacteria and parasites in the water, which have to be treated with chemicals before it is safe to drink.

Most tap water is recycled, probably numerous times in larger cities, and contains recycled oestrogens and other hormones, from the contraceptive pill and unwanted pharmaceutical drugs that are flushed down the toilet,[9] as well as pesticides and other toxic compounds such as cadmium, barium and mercury.[10] Every time you drink, you could be adding small amounts of toxins to your system that may affect your health.[11] Be aware and check your water out.

TEST YOUR WATER

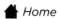 *Home*

There are inexpensive water-testing kits, such as WaterSafe, available on the Internet, which will give you an idea of how safe your water is to drink.

TOP TIP

The ZeroWater filter jug, available online, does just what it says – reduces the toxins in the water to zero. Inexpensive but incredibly effective, it also comes with a water-testing kit so that you can test your tap water (zerowater.co.uk).

Still thirsty

If you're always thirsty, your mouth is dry and your lips feel cracked, however much water you drink then something isn't working properly. It may not be how much water you are taking in, but how well it is being utilized by your body,[12] and sometimes this is due to prescription medications. Drugs for heart disease, stomach ulcers and depression can all alter your thirst mechanism, and certain diseases do the same – diabetes being the major culprit. Old age also brings with it the same problem. Sometimes the issue lies with the kidneys, because diabetes and high blood pressure can affect how they function, as can an infection or kidney stones, and you may need a couple of acupuncture sessions to strengthen your kidney meridian.

If your eyes are also dry, this can indicate a nutritional deficiency. Drink as much as possible and supplement with magnesium, B vitamins and fish oils to resolve the problem. If you drink more water than most people, but often feel light-headed and tired or have low blood pressure, you may be low in vasopressin. This hormone is secreted by the pituitary gland and keeps the body from losing too much water by increasing the amount that is reabsorbed by the kidneys. Increasing your salt intake at mealtimes and drinking less water should resolve it. If this doesn't work, consult your doctor, who may need to give you an intravenous sodium chloride infusion to get you back on track.

Action plan

→ **Be aware:** Work out how much and what you're drinking, and then increase the amount of water if necessary. Men should drink around 3 litres (6 pints) a day; women approximately 2 litres (4$1/4$ pints).

→ **Drink often:** Keep a bottle of water on your desk, in your car or close at hand at all times. Half the problem is that we simply forget to drink. Top yourself up by drinking small glasses regularly throughout the day.

→ **Avoid plastic:** If you regularly buy bottled water, choose glass bottles where possible, as plastic bottles contain phthalates that can leach chemicals into your water.

TOP TIPS

- *The Sippo smart cup and app can help to keep you properly hydrated, keeping tabs on how much you drink each day and reminding you if your water levels go down (sippo.com).*

- *If you find it hard to drink even a couple of glasses of water a day, then The Right Cup might be the solution. This specially designed cup comes in berry, orange, apple, peach, cola and grape flavours, and cleverly tricks your brain into thinking that plain drinking water is flavoured. With no sugar or artificial sweeteners, this could be the health invention of the century (therightcup.com).*

➔ **Supplement:** Dr Patrick Flanagan's MegaHydrate is a dietary supplement that increases hydration. Its benefits have been demonstrated in a number of studies.[13]

➔ **Eat more high-water foods:** Cucumbers, celery, lettuce, watermelon and most fruits and vegetables tend to be low in calories and high in nutrients. Approximately 20 per cent of your daily water intake comes from the food you eat.

Magnetize your water

Some studies suggest that drinking water that has been treated with magnets can prevent the build-up of plaque in your arteries, act as a diuretic to reduce water retention, bloating and puffiness, and improve digestion. Another study found that it prevents hair greying, reduces pH acidity and rebalances female hormones,[14] and also affects the blood and repairs DNA damage.[15] Russian hospitals use magnetized water to dissolve stones in the bladder and the kidneys painlessly.[16–18]

MAGNETIZE YOUR WATER

🌿 *Remedy*

Buy two magnets, with each side clearly marked either north or south. Make sure they are at least 3,000 MGO. Take a glass bottle of water and place it between the two magnets – with the south pole of one magnet facing the north pole of the other. Leave the water for 24 hours and then drink it within three to four days. Keep the bottle of magnetized water at room temperature, not in the fridge.

Chapter 21

Stand Tall: Fitness Facts

'Those who think they have no time for exercise
will sooner or later have to find time for illness.'

EDWARD STANLEY

Are you one of those people who has every intention of exercising, but can't quite stick to it? Do you make that New Year's resolution to join the gym, pay a fortune to make sure you're committed but then fail to put in more than a handful of appearances? Your yoga membership is inclusive and fully paid up, but three visits was enough? The voice inside your head says, 'We'll go tomorrow – there are much more important things to do today.' Despite your best efforts, does exercise just not seem to be for you?

And yet we all know that we really, really need to do it, because being active helps to maintain both physical and emotional health.[1] Regular exercise maintains physical strength, boosts circulation and improves the removal of toxins. Exercise also aids digestion, opens up your arteries, strengthens the heart and regulates blood pressure; it has even been shown to slow the effects of ageing and helps to avoid many age-related diseases, including Alzheimer's, osteoporosis, heart disease and diabetes.[2] Regular exercise improves your state of mind and feelings of wellbeing,[3] and has been shown to be as effective as CBT or antidepressants. Finally, exercise also decreases the effects of stress, reducing elevated stress hormones.[4]

Exercise is definitely one of the most important things you can do to help yourself stay healthy. But exercise is also all about balance. Too little and your body weakens and gets congested – too much and you are in danger of wearing out your adrenals.

There are classes to suit all tastes, everything from gentler forms of exercise such as yoga and Pilates to rebounding, Zumba and spinning. Go to your local health club or gym or look online and choose something that appeals. Set yourself an exercise target (i.e. 40 minutes three times a week or 20 minutes' five times a week) and, if possible, aim for a combination of aerobic exercise (e.g. dance or running), stretching exercise (e.g. yoga, pilates, tai chi) and resistance training (e.g. weights, lifting). You should come out of your class feeling energized and revitalized, not tired and shattered. Overdoing it defeats the purpose.

TOP TIP

Running has well-documented health benefits. It combines both resistance and aerobic exercise, and has positive mental benefits to boot.[5]

But if just thinking about exercise makes you groan, then look for something new that will actually add to your day and is fun. Something you look forward to is easier to commit to than something you dread. Try belly dancing, ballroom dancing, Bollywood or street dancing – try something that you have always meant to do but never got around to.

Something is very much better than nothing[6] and even 20 minutes of fast walking three times a week is sufficient provided it increases your heart rate. Walk to the shops instead of getting in your car. Walk up the stairs to your office instead of taking the lift. Get off the bus a few stops earlier and walk. Remember what activities you used to enjoy as a child, perhaps roller or ice skating, hockey or football, and then find a suitable class or group to join. If it's close to where you live, you may find it easier to incorporate into your daily routine. And if you're still struggling to get motivated to exercise then consider a session of hypnotherapy to help you feel more positive about it. The bottom line? Do whatever you can, but don't overdo it. Too much exercise can stress you more than strengthen.[7]

FITNESS FORENSICS TEST

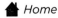 Home

Make a note of how often you:

- Do cardiovascular exercise, where your heart rate is elevated for a period of time and you feel slightly out of breath? How many times per week and for how many minutes?

- How many times per week and for how many minutes do you stretch or have a yoga or Pilates practice?

- How many times per week and for how long do you do resistance training?

SIT-AND-REACH TEST

🏠 *Home*

This is a common measure of the flexibility and suppleness of your lower back and hamstrings. You'll need a ruler and, if possible, another person to mark down the result.

1. Sit on the floor with your legs stretched out straight in front of you, shoes off.

2. Put the soles of your feet flat against a step or box. Both knees should be locked and pressed flat to the floor, and you can help by holding them down.

3. Put the ruler on the step, with the 0 end pointing towards you.

4. With your palms facing down, hands flat out in front of you, reach forwards along the ruler as far as you can.

5. After some practice reaches, reach forwards without overstraining and hold that position for one to two seconds while the measurement is recorded. Be sure to stay still and not make any jerky movements.

6. Record your score to the nearest centimetre as the distance reached by your hands.

Understanding your results

Very flexible is 20–30cm (8–12in) over your toes. Average is anything over 10cm (4in) over your toes and poor is anything less than 8cm (3in), where 0 is your toes themselves. If you find yourself in the 'poor' section, even five minutes a day of simple stretching exercises will get you more flexible in a week or so.

AEROBIC FITNESS TEST

🏠 *Home*

You learned how to measure your pulse rate in Chapter 1, and this is a good way to assess your exercise recovery time and an accurate measure of your fitness.

1. Check and record your pulse in your notebook (see Chapter 1, page 23). Time it over a minute.

2. Take a brisk 1.5km (1 mile) walk. You can do the walk anywhere, outside or on a track, or on a treadmill. After you complete the walk, check your watch and record the time it took you to finish, in minutes and seconds, in your notebook.

3. Then check and record your pulse once more. Your heart rate is a measure of your aerobic fitness.

As you increase the amount of exercise you take, you will quickly see an improvement in both time and heart rate, so keep a note as a way to chart your improving health over the next few months.

ABDOMINAL 'CORE STRENGTH' TEST

🏠 *Home*

Being able to hold a strong plank position is a good way to test your core stability (the strength of your deepest abdominal muscles, those that wrap around your torso and support your spine). When your core is weak, it has a negative impact on your posture and makes injury far more likely.

1. Get into a plank position, with your body in a straight line, weight supported on your forearms and flexed toes. Your elbows should be bent, hands resting forwards or clasped in front of you.

2. Pull your belly button towards your spine to engage your deep abdominal muscles. See how long you can maintain this position, without overstraining or compensating by arching your back in either direction. You should feel your core muscles working and may shake a little.

3. A fit man should be able to hold the plank position for just shy of two minutes. A fit woman should be able to manage one minute, 30 seconds.

Never continue to hold this position when you feel you have lost control or you could injure your back. Build up your practice gradually by increasing the amount of time you hold it for incrementally.

TOP TIP

There are loads of fitness and workout apps. Try Fitness Blender, an online exercise class that offers more than 400 free workout videos (fitnessblender.com) or the app MyFitnessPal.

Action plan

➔ **Make a commitment to exercise more:** Choose your preferred activity and then pay in advance for an entire course. If you have already spent the money you are much less likely to 'waste' it and miss the class.

→ **One-to-one:** If you can, have a few one-to-one sessions with a personal trainer. That way you do it right, right from the start, and your routine quickly becomes automatic, boosting your confidence and upping your chances of sticking with it. Alternatively, find a buddy to exercise with, so you can support and motivate each other.

→ **Encourage yourself:** Encouraging yourself with silent positive statements like 'You can do this', 'Feeling great' and 'Pushing through' have been shown to trigger biochemical changes in the body that can improve your ability to exercise.[8]

→ **Build a playlist that inspires you and listen to it each time you exercise:** If you love the music, you will associate great feelings with exercising and look forward to your sessions.

→ **If you just can't:** If you really, really can't exercise, for whatever reason, then check out inmindinbody.com. It has a series of strength-training MP3s based on the concept that the mind can condition the body, and that visualized exercise can be nearly as effective as doing the real thing, making you quantifiably physically stronger. Amazingly, it really works.

Caring for your body

Along with exercise, taking care of your posture can really improve your physical, mental and emotional wellbeing. We often end up spending way too much time sitting at our computers, driving long distances, slumped on sofas and hunched over desks. Over time, poor posture can compress your internal organs, triggering aches and pains, and making your heart and lungs work even harder. If even one area is out of alignment, the rest of the body has to alter itself to compensate. This can add additional stress to already overworked muscles and the result is pain, often leading to muscle or joint injury and frequent headaches.

Bad posture can lead to back pain and a whopping 80 per cent of people suffer with back problems in their lifetime. In 2016, 8.8 million working days were lost owing to musculoskeletal problems.[9]

TEST HOW STRAIGHT YOU STAND

 Home

Stand in front of a mirror and look at your reflection. If you can draw a straight line from your earlobe through to your shoulders, hips and knees, and down to your middle ankles while standing in front of a mirror, then you have good posture.

Apps such as PostureZone will give you a benchmark to work from, analysing your weaknesses, improving your posture and allowing you to track improvement. You can also use the results to help you, and any trainer, develop a personalized workout that will strengthen rather than damage your body.

Stand tall

When your posture is good, it has a knock-on impact on all sorts of things: you breathe more deeply, you carry less tension in your muscles, your digestive system is able to function better. Realigning your posture, and working on the way you sit, stand and move, can have a powerful impact on your health.[10] If you have poor posture, then consider seeing a chiropractor or an osteopath, who can adjust your spine while releasing muscle stress. McTimoney chiropractic is a less well known but particularly gentle and effective form of manipulation to try, while the Alexander Technique is another method for retraining your posture. Exercise can help too.

Pilates and yoga both strengthen the upper back and shoulders, as well as the core abdominal muscles that support your spine, offering an effective and inexpensive way to improve posture. Regular stretching will also improve your stance.

TOP TIP

Rolfing, a technique used by many ballet dancers, is a therapy that works on your body structure muscle by muscle, moving it back into position. Once realigned, the body seems to recognize the corrected positions and retains them, releasing you to sit straight and walk tall.

Poor posture has an effect on the mind and the reverse is equally true: happy, successful people tend to stand firm and upright. Depressed and anxious people seem to turn in on themselves, slouching with rounded shoulders. Research from Columbia and Harvard universities demonstrated that how we stand can also affect our decision-making subconsciously, and can make us feel more powerful and in control of life. Standing tall in an expansive pose quantifiably improved the feeling of power and control, and also made that person 45 per cent more likely to take a risky bet. Expansive postures also have physical benefits, altering hormone levels, lowering cortisol and upping testosterone levels, which in turn protects from disease.[11]

TOP TIP

Avoid wearing clothes that are too tight – jeans or belts, for instance – as they can throw off the body's alignment. High-heeled shoes are to be avoided as they shift your weight forwards onto the balls of the feet, forcing the body to realign itself to compensate for the change. Too large or too tight shoes create structural problems by similarly skewing the body.

Also, did you know that sitting for a long period of time causes your energy levels to fall and your mood to change, so that you're more likely to get tired and irritable? Studies have shown that slouching while moving also increases feelings of depression and lowers energy levels.[12] Your memory and thinking abilities depend on an adequate flow of blood from your heart to your brain, and poor posture can restrict this flow and lower concentration levels, often contributing to a feeling of mind fog.

Similarly, changing your thoughts and feelings can change the way your body holds itself. Do one, then try the other, and see what works for you. Once you become aware of poor habits it is much easier to change them. However, changing bad habits takes focus and concentration, and repetition of the new stance until it becomes automatic for the body.

Action plan

➜ **Make simple changes:** Check the position of your chair in relation to your computer and ensure you aren't rounding your shoulders or tilting your chin forwards to look at your screen. And don't cradle your phone under your chin.

➜ **Alternate:** Try not to carry your handbag, laptop bag, child or shopping on the same side of your body. Alternate hands, hips and sides. Check that you don't always put your weight on the same leg.

→ **Tuck in:** Don't stand with your bottom sticking out. Consciously pull it in to correct it and avoid lower back strain.

→ **Take regular breaks:** Sitting for long periods (even a long commute with your shoulders hunched as you tap e-mails into your smartphone) can lead to neck and upper-back tension. Get up, do a quick stretch and walk around for a while.

→ **Walk tall:** Walking with a book balanced on your head or imagining a piece of string attached to the top of your head, pulling you gently upwards towards the sky, can realign your spine, neck and shoulders, and help you to stand straight and tall.

→ **Invest in an ergonomic chair:** This will keep you sitting upright at your desk. Alternatively, swap sitting for standing and invest in a standing desk.

→ **Do some exercise:** Strengthening your core – the abdominal and lower back muscles that connect to your spine and pelvis – is one of the best ways to improve posture.

→ **Correct poor posture:** Book some sessions with a bodywork therapist who can realign you. Rolfing and the Alexander Technique can both reverse the effects of bad standing habits in a few sessions.

Chapter 22

Stress: The Hidden Menace

*'The part can never be well
unless the whole is well.'*

PLATO

Stress isn't something that we simply experience when we're under pressure at work or home. It has many other faces and its effects on our wellbeing are far-reaching. Stress is there in a body that's undernourished and short on sleep. It's the reason why some people get one cold after another, or why they've learned to live with bloating and stomach cramps, or the explanation for constant brain fog.

IDENTIFY STRESS

 Home

To help you to identify whether or not you're suffering from hidden stress, read through the 12 most common symptoms and see how many apply to you:[1]

1.   You're constantly tired and regularly wake up exhausted.

2. You suffer from bloating, stomach cramps, constipation or the runs, or have been diagnosed with IBS (irritable bowel syndrome).

3. You have a low libido.

4. Your appetite is disordered: either you're constantly hungry, craving sugary foods, or you've lost your appetite.

5. You struggle to sleep well. You might find it difficult to drop off, or wake up in the middle of the night, worrying, and find it difficult to get back to sleep.

6. You've put on weight and can't seem to shift it.

7. You suffer from repeated colds and poor immunity, and have come to accept feeling generally under the weather as par for the course.

8. Your mind feels foggy, and you find it difficult to focus on work and conversation.

9. You are anxious and may suffer panic attacks or feel consumed by worry.

10. You suffer constant discomfort and aches in your joints or muscles.

11. You experience regular headaches or migraines.

12. You have a bad back that keeps flaring up.

Obviously, depending on the severity of symptoms, you may well need to pay your doctor a visit for help. The advice in this book is designed to work in tandem with conventional medical treatment. But I passionately believe that it's important to treat the cause not the symptom and if you're experiencing any combination of the aforementioned, it's vital to invest time and care into identifying the source of your stress, so that you can then reset the balance at a deep level.

CORTISOL TEST

✚ *Doctor*

> The best way to measure your levels of cortisol, the stress hormone, is with a saliva test, where samples are taken four times in a 24-hour period to analyse the levels of cortisol in your system and identify how your adrenals are functioning (see Chapter 13, page 113).

Stress and your immune system

Your immune system works 24/7 to keep you well. During the day, it protects you against external invaders – bacteria, viruses and germs. At night as you sleep, it gets on with various repair jobs, fighting any internal battles that need to be won, releasing natural killer cells to attack cancer cells or calming inflammation.

The impact of too much stress on your immune system is huge,[2] as it alters your biochemistry and stops all sorts of processes working properly. Stress affects the functioning of your brain and the clarity of your thinking. It's not just difficult emotional life events that cause stress – work or family issues, divorce, moving home, financial problems or the death of someone close to you – but a build-up of the stress is going on inside you too. Each time you eat too much, every vitamin or mineral that your body is struggling to manage without, or is overloaded with, every toxin you eat or chemical you breathe in adds to your stress levels, until your immune system stops working properly.

The systems and organs that make up the immune system include:

- Hormones

- Antibodies

- White blood cells

- Bone marrow

- Spleen

- Lymphatic system

- Thymus

- Tonsils

- Liver

- Appendix

Emotional stress

The mind and the body are inextricably linked. Clean up your body and your mental issues will often resolve. Clear your thoughts and emotions, and physical ailments will often disappear. It is hard to overstate the importance of sorting your mental and emotional 'stuff'.

You may not think you have any unresolved emotional problems causing you stress, but look closely again. Very few of us escape emotional trauma of some kind. Have you dealt with any of the grief, loss, anger or betrayal that life so often throws our way by burying them deep inside you? Swallowed the pain and locked it away?

Loss of something or someone can cause huge trauma that sends shock waves through your body at every level and dozens of studies show that emotional stress compromises immunity,[3] whilst a major trauma such as a divorce, bereavement or PTSD has been proven to have a negative effect on everything from heart health to Alzheimer's risk.[4]

Just like physical stress, emotional stress places huge strain on your immune system. Suppressing negative emotions and traumatic memories year after year can slowly drain your energy, eventually overwhelming you and affecting your health. It can happen gradually over a series of years or in one fell swoop, like a tidal wave that brings down everything before it.

Healing emotional stress

Emotional healing doesn't happen overnight, but starting to address any issues is the pathway to healing and there are only two initial steps to emotional health:

1. Identify any unresolved issues.

2. Find a counsellor or trained professional to help you work through them.

You can take a traditional approach, such as seeing a psychiatrist or psychologist, or a less conventional one and work with a therapist or life coach. Both work, but I recommend investigating all the options. Read the articles 'How to choose a therapist to work with' and 'Alternative ways to unburden your mind' at ReBoot Health (reboothealth.co.uk) for an in-depth overview. But most important of all, spend time finding the right therapist for you, so that you feel comfortable with your choice. That decision will play a huge part in your therapy's success.

Breathe – let it all go...

Breathing is a core part of the practice of yoga and has measurable health benefits. It calms the body and the mind. Lots of studies have demonstrated the benefits of yogic breathing, showing that it can have a positive impact on everything from stress and depression to blood pressure.[5]

Even without considering these impressive benefits, breathing deeply and in a focused way can stop your mind's endless chatter and halt negative thinking, allowing you to connect deeply and peacefully with yourself. Highly stressed people tend to take only shallow breaths most of the time (see Chapter 2, page 34 for the CP test), but deep yogic breathing floods your cells with oxygen, and gives your body additional energy to get rid of toxins, renew organs and generally feel better. It calms the 'fight or flight' response that puts your nervous system on edge, and reduces stress and anxiety.

DEEP BREATHING

🍃 *Remedy*

Lie flat on your back and make sure you are comfortable and warm. Place a pillow or a folded towel under your knees and relax your whole body. Put your hand over your tummy button and feel your stomach rise slowly up and down as you breathe gently in and out. Notice how your breath feels. Is it shallow? Is it ragged or uneven? Try to make your breathing as calm and smooth as possible.

Breathe in through your nose and out through your mouth. Gently fill your body with air, drawing your breath deep into your stomach. Pause slightly after you finish each breath.

Feel how your stomach expands and contracts with each breath in and out.

Try to take a deeper breath in, hold it a little longer and then slowly breathe out before repeating the process. Do this for 8-10 breaths and notice how much calmer you feel. The more slowly and deeply you breathe, the calmer you will become. Your body will be benefitting from increased levels of oxygen and your mind from the unaccustomed stillness.

TOP TIP

If you need help with the practice, the Breathe Deep app makes it all very simple to do regularly, and offers a choice of yogic breathing techniques. Headspace, an online meditation app, offers guided meditation and mindfulness techniques to get you started.

Action plan

➔ **Eat well:** Vitamin B complex and foods rich in B vitamins will help to balance and calm your brain chemistry and neurotransmitters, while calcium and magnesium can help you to relax and sleep. Eat healthy fats too, as these can reduce inflammation and calm your mind. (See also Chapter 19 and the Appendix.)

➔ **Mindfulness meditation:** Deep breathing and stilling the mind have been found to reduce anxiety and improve the immune system's response to stress.[6] Try the Calm app to get into a daily routine.

→ **Exercise:** Getting active releases endorphins that can improve mood and reduce stress. Exercise also helps to regulate your blood sugar levels and sleep cycle. (See also Chapters 19 and 23.)

→ **Book in for acupuncture:** This ancient practice regulates the nervous system and affects all your different systems, releasing, balancing and calming stress in the process.

→ **Get referred:** Ask your doctor to refer you for a course of cognitive behavioural therapy (CBT), which has been proven to lower anxiety and stress by helping you to reframe the way you think about events in your life, reducing stress in the process.

→ **Visit a medical herbalist:** Holy basil, ginseng, ashwagandha, maca and rhodiola can all help the body manage stress by regulating hormones and calming the system. A qualified herbalist can tailor the dose to your requirements.

→ **Essential oils:** Lavender, myrrh, frankincense and bergamot can reduce inflammation, improve immunity, balance hormones and help you sleep. Invest in a diffuser and breathe them in while you work or sleep.

TOP TIP

PAUSE is a relaxation app that is said to reduce stress levels. You follow a changing blob of light around the screen with your finger and the action actively moves your mind into the present moment – mindfulness at your fingertip!

DESIGN YOUR OWN 'OFF' SWITCH

🦋 *Remedy*

Feeling stressed triggers the 'fight or flight' response causing stress hormones to flood your body (see Chapter 13, page 110). In today's stressful world, that 'switch' is often continually on, leaving little in your reserves for a true emergency. You may feel you are running on close to empty right now, but you can quickly get control back and calm your body's responses by designing your own off-switch.

1. Imagine that you can see your 'fight or flight' switch. Notice where it is in your body, exactly what it looks like – shape, size, what it's made of, and which way it switches 'off' and 'on'.

2. Consciously switch it off now. Imagine yourself pressing or turning it off and notice how your body immediately relaxes.

3. In your mind's eye, see the hormones retreating, your body slowing all its reactions, and connect a feeling of calm and peace to the whole image.

4. If you use diaphragmatic breathing at the same time (see Chapter 22, page 212), which signals to your brain that everything is OK, you will get a double dose of calm.

When the next stressful thing happens to you, even if it is relatively unimportant, your switch will switch itself on automatically, out of habit, again releasing cortisol, adrenaline and noradrenaline to help you get through the situation. Just make sure that afterwards you take a few seconds to switch it off again consciously. In time, it will become automatic.

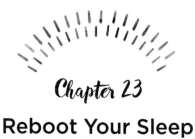

Chapter 23

Reboot Your Sleep

'Sleep is that golden chain that ties our health and our bodies together.'

THOMAS DEKKER

No one really knows all the reasons why we sleep or precisely what we do when we're sleeping. We do know that the body uses the time to repair and rebalance its systems. The increasing stresses of everyday living, however, means that more and more people struggle to sleep, and are not getting the rest and repair time they need. The 24-hour cycle that regulates your sleep pattern, often referred to as your body clock, working optimally is an essential part of getting well. If you can't sleep, you can't function and life can become hard to bear.

Everybody is different, but most of us need six to nine hours a night and recent research seems to indicate that around seven hours is optimal,[1] although this is hotly debated. However, experts do agree that it is sleep quality that counts rather than the number of hours spent asleep. As well as impacting your health,[2] your sleep quality is also a barometer of your state of mind and wellbeing.

KEEP A SLEEP LOG

 Home

For three nights, spaced out over a week or so, keep a notebook by your bed. First thing in the morning, make a note of the following:

- Estimated time it took you to get to sleep.

- Number of hours between falling asleep and waking up (how much sleep you've had).

- Did you wake up in the night? If so, at what time and how often, and how easily did you get back to sleep?

- Did you wake up naturally or artificially (i.e. alarm)?

- How did you feel when you woke up?

Keeping a note of your sleep state now and in a few weeks' time is a helpful marker of your progress.

Restore your circadian rhythm

Your ability to sleep depends on your circadian rhythm[3] – the 24-hour body clock that makes you wake up in the morning and feel sleepy as night approaches. The clock is activated by light, which signals that it's time to get up or go to bed.

The longer you're awake, the greater your need for sleep – but if your clock isn't set properly, you just won't be able to. Jetlag, for example, is the result of moving into a different time zone without adjusting your clock. When jetlag sets in, you can reset your body clock by looking at the sun (not directly or you could damage your eyes!).

Recent research also shows that the time you eat your meals can affect your circadian rhythm.[4] Fixed, consistent eating routines help you to sleep, but changing your usual pattern and eating later can throw off your body clock and ability to sleep. Exercise, hormones, temperature and caffeine can all affect your sleep patterns, too, but light is the most powerful regulator. Bright light stimulates the pineal gland in the brain, creating serotonin, which keeps you happy and wakeful. Darkness, on the other hand, triggers melatonin, which makes you sleepy.

The light bulb is probably responsible for many of our sleep problems today – suppressing melatonin levels and keeping us wakeful far past our natural sleep times. Checking e-mails, watching your favourite late-night comedian or replying to a text message in bed seems harmless enough, but the sleep disruption caused by these light-emitting devices is significant.

Circadian rhythm is affected by the colour of the light – for instance, the blue light in the colour spectrum tells your brain it's day and time to wake up – and by the intensity of the light, whether that is inside or outside. Go outside for 30 minutes in the morning to wake up your body. In Africa, where day and night comes regularly every 12 hours, the population's internal clocks work 12 hours on and 12 hours off, but in Europe it has been noted that the internal clocks shift as day and night waxes and wanes with the seasons. Putting the clocks backwards and forwards twice a year doesn't help.

Action plan

→ **Get your timings right:** If you struggle to fall asleep, make sure you consistently go to bed at the same time every night, preferably before 11 p.m. Research shows that three hours' sleep loss is the equivalent of a 50 per cent reduction in your immune system's efficiency, so consistent late nights are a no-no.[5]

→ **Create some pre-bed sleep rituals:** Do the same thing every night before you go to sleep. Just like letting a baby know that it's night time by following the same routine at the same time each evening, do the same thing for your mind. Perhaps have a warm bath with sleep-inducing lavender oil, listen to the same music or lie in bed and do a relaxation exercise. Hot baths help you sleep because your body has to drop its core temperature to get rid of the excess heat from the water, which makes you drowsy. Watching a violent movie and then expecting your mind to chill is not going to work, nor is reading a gripping book before you turn out the lights.

→ **Follow good sleep hygiene practices:**

- Make your bedroom a calm, clear, restful place for sleeping.

- Remove computers, laptops, phones and other devices from the bedroom, as the electromagnetic stress can stimulate rather than calm.[6]

- Sunlight at the 'wrong' time affects the body clock, so make sure your bedroom is properly dark at night. Put in blackout blinds if you need to.

- A cool temperature is best, because your body releases melatonin at lower temperatures – ideally 16–18°C (61–64°F).[7] If it's too hot your body can't rest. Open the windows or turn down the heating.

- If traffic or noisy neighbours keep you awake at night, have a fan whirring in the background to create an even white noise that cuts out background disturbance.

~ Is your mattress comfortable? Even something as seemingly minor as a lumpy pillow can repeatedly disturb your rest, so update your bedding if necessary.

TOP TIPS

- *The Beddit (beddit.com) is a sleep sensor that monitors your breathing, movement and sleep cycles, and lets you track your sleeping habits over time so you can see what makes a difference to the quality of your sleep.*

- *If you wake yourself up by twitching in the night, try soaking in a bath of Epsom salts before going bed. The magnesium sulphate sinks into your muscles, relaxing them. Don't use Epsom salts if you are pregnant or breastfeeding, have high blood pressure or cardiovascular problems.*

➜ **Don't eat and drink late at night:** Eating a heavy meal late in the evening can also affect sleep. The body has to use all its energy to digest the food and sleep stops that process, leaving both sleeping and digesting working less than perfectly.

➜ **Avoid alcohol and caffeine:** Alcohol and caffeine are not only stimulants, but also cause dehydration so can cause you to wake up in the night with a dry mouth and headache.[8] Try cutting out both out for a few days and see if that makes a difference to your sleep.

➜ **Drink herbal tea:** Camomile or valerian[9] can help you to relax before bed.

➜ **Eat sleep-making foods:** Try a few days of easily digested foods at night – salads, fruit and vegetables. Bananas trigger the production of melatonin, and oatcakes, honey and Marmite are also good. Warm oat milk with nutmeg contains tryptophan, which raises your levels of serotonin (the 'sleep' chemical). A recent study of omega-3 fish oil taken at night added an additional hour to the participants' sleep totals.[10] Cherry juice also helps with insomnia.[11] Try these remedies one at a time and notice which one helps you get better-quality rest.

→ **Try a sleep supplement:** Experiment with the following supplements one at a time to see which one works for you. Take three capsules of L-tryptophan (500mg) in half a glass of orange juice before bed. Tryptophan seems to work better for women with sleep problems – melatonin for men. Time-release melatonin helps you go to sleep and also keeps you sleeping calmly through the night.[12] Liposomal spray melatonin is also useful for preventing jetlag.

TOP TIPS

- *Blue-blocking glasses take the blue light out of the spectrum so that you can read in the evening and still manage to drift off to sleep (blublocker.com). Ocushield is a clear filter developed by an optician that you can stick invisibly on the front of your iPad or phone that also cuts out blue light and prevents sleep disturbance (ocushield.com).*

- *If you have problems getting to sleep or waking up in the morning, the Lumie® Bodyclock Starter 30 is a light that works both as an alarm and night time wind-down. It slowly fades or brightens over a period of 30 minutes, allowing your body clock to adjust easily to the process of waking or sleeping (lumie.com).*

- *If you want to see exactly where your body clock is going wrong, the FitSleep, a small square box that attaches to your phone (fitsleep.net), will give you minute-by-minute statistics on how you spend the night – heart rate, breathing, body movements – and then transmits alpha waves for longer, deeper sleep.*

Stress and sleep

If you're heavily stressed, then all of the aforementioned will only work to a partial degree. Spend time working out how you can resolve the issues and don't shoulder the burdens alone. We often think if we can't hold it all together, the world will fall apart, but usually the opposite is true. Whether you talk to friends or take professional advice, make sure you address the issues rather than hoping they will just go away. (See also Chapter 22.)

Action plan

→ **Write it down:** Every night, before you go to sleep, write a list of the things your brain is struggling with. Once they are written down, your mind doesn't then need to bring them to your attention continually and wake you repeatedly in the night to make sure you haven't forgotten them. Try it – it really works!

→ **Experiment with different complementary therapies:** Acupuncture has been found to help with sleep problems. Use it to strengthen your bladder meridian. Hypnotherapy can calm mental stress and worry associated with too little sleep and reset broken sleep patterns. Emotional Freedom Technique (EFT) is also effective at resolving underlying issues.

➜ **Give yourself a break:** Having trouble unwinding at night is often connected to being too wired up in the day. The body gets used to being continually on the go, so you may need to change your daily pattern. Make sure you take a lunch break, rather than working through it. Read a book, go for a leisurely stroll – let your mind know it can chill, that this is your time. Don't spend the time doing e-mails – just be peaceful. Doze off for a few minutes if you have somewhere you can. Even a 15-minute nap can relax and calm the system, and give you a burst of renewed energy to continue with your day. Leave work behind you when you walk out of the door in the evening. If you simply can't, then set fixed times at home to focus on it – and stick to those timings. Get into a habit of setting boundaries and your body will find it easier to relax at bedtime.

➜ **Relax and breathe:** Try placing your hand on your stomach, and focus your mind on how your belly moves slowly up and down as you breathe in and out. Whenever your mind starts to drift away and think about other things, bring it back to those rhythmic movements and you will find yourself asleep before you know it.

How do you sleep?

Your sleeping position can also affect how rested you feel in the morning, whether you have any joint pain and whether you snore.

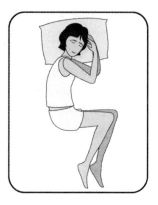

The foetus

This is the most popular of all the sleep positions and the way 51 per cent of all women sleep. Sleeping on your side keeps your spine elongated, and reduces neck and back pain; it also reduces snoring and acid reflux.

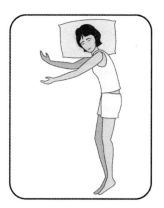

The yearner

The yearner is a good position for your back muscles and ligaments. Less stress for the discs in the spine, but hard on the neck – 13 per cent of us sleep like this.

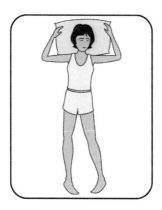

The starfish

The starfish is likely to make you snore but is good for minimizing back and neck pain. The starfish reduces acid reflux and is one of the few positions that leaves you less wrinkled from not squishing your face into the pillow. It doesn't squash your breasts either.

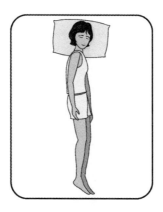

The log

Only 15 per cent of us sleep in the log position, but it keeps your spine straight and unstressed; it's bad for wrinkles but good for snoring less.

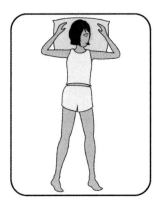

The freefall

Chosen by only 7 per cent of us, sleeping on your stomach puts pressure on the neck and joints. The freefall position is also hard on the back, as you don't receive any support under the curve of your spine. Freefall is however good for digestion and not snoring, but keeping your neck twisted at 90 degrees can cause pain and numbness in the morning.

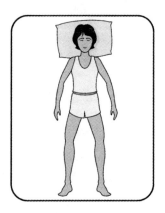

The soldier

The soldier position is preferred by 8 per cent of us, but it is the most likely to make you snore and comes with a high risk of sleep apnoea. Again, this position is good for acid reflux, as well as back and neck pain.

TOP TIP

Subscribe to reboothealth.co.uk and receive a free 30-page sleep e-book.

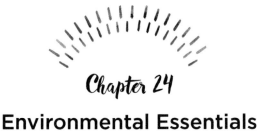

Chapter 24

Environmental Essentials

'It's the environment, stupid!'

BRUCE LIPTON

So far we've focused on the body, but in this final chapter I'd like you to consider your external environment and become aware of how it can affect your wellbeing.

Toxic home

Did you know that if you clean your home with chemical supermarket sprays, use lotions and potions on your body and hair, and wear synthetic clothes that it's easy to build up toxicity unknowingly from everyday items?

More than 3,000 different chemicals are used to make cleaning products, toiletries, make-up, hairspray, sun creams, body lotions, perfume, and shower and bath gels. Household cleaners, sprays and polishes all contain chemicals that build up in the human body over time, and can slow down its systems and functions.[1] Residues from plastics in bottles, pesticides and detergents mimic hormones, blocking oestrogen or progesterone, and can cause havoc with the adrenal and thyroid glands.[2-3] Even cotton wool tampons, toilet paper and nappies all contain chlorinated bleach.

Unless you go and live in the woods then it's very difficult to avoid all these products, but there are some simple changes you can make to reduce your toxic load. Start by being aware of what's in your shopping bag by checking labels and buying organic, natural products whenever you can. Most household cleaning products can be made inexpensively and naturally. Recipes often use vinegar, lemon juice or bicarbonate of soda and were used safely by households for hundreds of years, right up to the last few decades.

Health check your home

All of the following chemicals have been found to have negative health consequences on our wellbeing, so avoid the following when you can:

Bisphenol A (BPA): A synthetic oestrogen used in the manufacture of some plastic products, in the linings of tins, in retail receipts and more. BPA is not always listed on labels and passes quickly into the body, where it causes hormonal disruption and cancer. Breast cancer charities have called for its removal from all food products.[4-6]

PVC and vinyl: Found in soft plastic toys, shower curtains and flooring. PVC and vinyl have been found to be carcinogenic, so opt for PVC-free products wherever possible.[7]

Formaldehyde: Found in building products, such as composite flooring, chipboard and ply board, formaldehyde is carcinogenic and can trigger respiratory problems, as well as irritate the skin, eyes, nose and throat.[8]

Triclosan: Found in antibacterial soaps and products and absorbed through your skin, triclosan affects hormones and weakens the immune system.[9]

Phthalates: Used in the manufacture of plastic bottles and cosmetic plastics, phthalates can have a disruptive effect on hormones and brain development.[10] Many cosmetics and bottled liquids are now labelled phthalate-free, so check the labels before buying.

1, 4-dioxane: Labelled as sodium lauryl sulphate and poly-ethylene glycol/PEG, this is a foaming agent used in many cosmetic and cleaning products; it can be harsh on the skin, cause headaches and drowsiness, and irritate the eyes, nose, throat and lungs.[11]

PFOA (Perfluorooctanoic acid): Found in nonstick pans and stain-resistant or treated fabrics, research studies indicate that PFOA may cause cancer.[12]

Parabens: Found in personal care products, including shampoos and lotions, as well as 90 per cent of many grocery products. Parabens are known to disrupt hormones, mimicking oestrogen by binding to receptors on the cells, triggering breast cell division and tumour growth. Research suggests small quantities are not harmful to health,[13] but long-term cumulative exposure can overload the body and trigger disease.

Action plan

→ **Garden safely:** Don't use chemical pesticides in your garden... ever.

→ **Cookware:** Use steel or cast-iron cookware and avoid nonstick pans.

→ **Avoid plastics when possible:** Avoid plastics numbered 3, 6 or 7. NEVER heat plastic in the microwave, dishwasher or sun, as it can cause endocrine-disrupting chemicals to leach into your food and drink.[14] Use a stainless steel reusable water bottle and store your food in glass; it's much safer.

→ **Avoid plug-in fragrances:** These contain phthalates and are best avoided. Use natural essential oils in a diffuser to keep your home smelling fresh and, if you buy a new car, keep the windows open until that 'new-car smell' (phthalates, again) is completely gone.

→ **Read labels:** Choose household products that do not have warnings of CAUTION, DANGER or CAUSTIC.

Clear your home

Along with keeping your home as toxin-free as possible, you can create a healthier home by making it as organized and clutter-free as possible. If you regularly come home to a sinkful of dirty dishes and piles of laundry, or overflowing shelves and cupboards, then perhaps it is time for a clear out.

Feng shui experts believe that your home is a reflection of what's going on inside you and small changes to your exterior environment can adjust your internal self – body and psyche – as well.[15] Imagine what might happen if you made large changes instead of small ones.

It doesn't have to be done all at once, but even a cupboard a month can result in bag loads of unwanted 'stuff', helping out the charity shop down the road. Recycle it all – let your rubbish become someone else's treasure and make your home a place you want to return to.

TOP TIP

If you suffer from headaches, visual problems or feeling sick, or if you just feel exhausted at the end of each day – whether at home or work – check for EMFs (electromagnetic fields) from nearby radio towers, Wi-Fi and electricity power lines. Electromagnetic radiation is invisible, but can be measured with an EMF meter, which you can rent or buy online. Test the fields given off by your phone, PC, washing machine and fridge, and scan the plugs by your bedside. Block the fields and you may resolve some of your health issues.

Heavy metals

The build-up of heavy metal deposits within the body – high levels of aluminium, copper, lead, arsenic or mercury – puts the immune system under huge strain.[16] We're exposed to heavy metals from a variety of sources, copper pipes, aluminium saucepans, mercury from dental fillings, fish and water, cosmetics, pesticides and the air that we breathe, but they are a disaster for the brain and may well be one of the triggers for developing Alzheimer's later in life.[17]

Symptoms of heavy metal overload can range from mild depression to bipolar disorder and personality changes, as well as muscle and joint pain, headaches, allergies and exhaustion. Heavy metals weaken your organs and affect most of the systems in the body.[18] Often, brain fog and memory problems are down to metal toxicity, so clear the metals and you may well clear your mind in the process.

TOXIC METALS TEST

✚ *Doctor*

A nutritionist or naturopathic doctor will be able to arrange a hair mineral analysis kit for you, which will identify whether or not metal toxicity is an issue. Or you can order a urine test online, which is then sent to a lab for analysis.

Action plan

→ **Detox:** Once you've identified the heavy metals, there are various products that can help eliminate them:

- ~ Chlorella, taken daily, binds with any metals and allows the body to excrete the toxins. You have to take 15–20 of the tiny pills a day (read the label for precise dosage) and expect to keep taking them for a year or so before testing again to check your progress.

- ~ PectaClear® is a researched heavy metal-removing formula with remarkable results.

- ~ Activated liquid zeolite is a liquid detox formula that removes heavy metals including mercury, cadmium, lead, arsenic, aluminium, tin and excess iron. It also removes radioactive metals such as strontium and caesium effectively. Take a few drops in water three times a day for between four to six weeks to detox your body (innovasion.com).

→ **Ask your naturopath to research chelation therapy with EDTA:** This chemical clears the whole system of toxins, pulling out heavy metals and all pollutants.

→ **Consult with a mercury-free dentist:** Only use an IAOMT mercury-safe dentist to have any amalgam fillings replaced. If your usual dentist offers to remove your fillings you may well end up in more trouble than leaving them in place. Specialist equipment and expertise is essential.

→ **Limit the amount of fish you eat:** Nearly all fish contains mercury and the bigger the fish, the more mercury, so aim for just two to three portions a week. Tuna, swordfish and marlin have the highest levels; lobster, skipjack tuna, cod, halibut, mahi-mahi and trout have medium levels; and salmon, herring, haddock, crab, clam, crayfish, pollock, perch, rainbow trout, sardines, shrimp and scallops the lowest.

→ **Sweat it out:** Find a far-infrared sauna and sweat the toxins out.

Mould

Many of us, and particularly anyone living in a damp home, will have high levels of mould in their surroundings. Some moulds are highly visible, as dark spots or damp patches on the bathroom walls for example, but they can also multiply out of sight, under the floor, around the edge of the bath and sink or behind water-using appliances. What you may not know is that mould can be toxic for your health, as the mould spores are released into the air, triggering allergies and compromising your immune system.

This is no big deal if you are fighting fit, but when your energy is low, mould exposure can weaken your body and change the way you think and feel. With 'push me pull you' tactics, mould spores overstimulate your immune system at the same time as blocking its ability to work properly, causing all kinds of physical and mental problems in the body.

If you have any of the following symptoms and have failed to resolve your problems, check for mould:

- Exhaustion

- Mood swings

- Difficulty concentrating, brain fog and memory issues

- Muscle cramps and aches

- Unexplained tiredness

- Headaches

- Persistent cough, asthma and sinus problems

- Itching

- Eye and throat irritation

ENVIRONMENTAL MOULD TEST

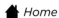 *Home*

> If you suspect that you have a mould allergy, you can test the levels of mould in your home with the online VCS (visual contrast sensitivity) test (vcstest.com), developed by Ken Hudnall from the US environmental agency. Mould can cause a reduction in contrast vision as it damages the nerve cells. Monitoring with the VCS test can tell you when you are clear of the infection.

MOULD IDENTIFICATION TEST

🏠 *Home*

If you are convinced you have a serious mould problem, there is a lab test called the ERMI that will identify the specific moulds causing your issues. ERMI stands for the Environmental Relative Moldiness Index. It is a US test and, based on the analysis of a single sample of dust from your home, can identify what moulds are affecting your health (emlab.com).

BLOOD TEST

✚ *Doctor*

Ask your doctor to do a blood test. Mould increases cytokine levels, which are a trigger for autoimmune diseases like rheumatism or lupus.

Once mould has established a presence, it is extremely difficult to remove, but it does need a combination of three things to grow – air, water and food (usually dust, wood or plasterboard) – and won't survive if you remove just one of them.

Action plan

→ **Clean it up:** There are all sorts of mould remedies, both natural and pharmaceutical, but if your health is noticeably affected, there is little point in doing less than a thorough attack on the spores.

~ Scrub the walls (wearing a facemask so you don't inhale even more spores) and, if necessary, repaint with anti-mould paint.

~ Find any damp or leaks and sort them.

~ Pull furniture back from the walls to allow the space to dry out.

~ Keep your home heated and well ventilated to avoid damp returning.

~ If after all that the mould still hasn't gone, you may need to call in the professionals to seal the room and heat-treat the problem.

TOP TIP

Bulletproof coffee is said to be the only coffee in the world especially developed to be resistant to mould. Created by Dave Asprey, it's a combination of coffee and MCT oil, which gives you a burst of energy, sharpens your brain and focuses your mind.

→ **Eat to mend the damage:** Have a green juice or a mug of hot water and apple cider vinegar each morning to alkalize your body, because mould hates an alkaline environment. Take a probiotic each day to wipe out the 'bad' bacteria in your gut. (See also Chapter 4.)

→ **Supplement and use herbs to boost your immunity:** Glutathione, omega-3 oils, vitamin D and artichoke leaf extract have all been shown to affect mould. Myrrhinil-Intest®, an antifungal made from chamomile flowers, birch charcoal and myrrh, absorbs the mould toxins internally via medically activated carbon and strengthens the immune system at the same time.

→ **Invest in an air purification system:** This can take out the spores and purify the air.

TOP TIPS

- *Diffuse myrrh or tea tree oil in a vaporizer in all your rooms. Myrrh is antimicrobial and will attack the mould toxins. Neat vinegar sprayed on the wall will kill around 82 per cent of mould spores.*

- *Download my e-book* Mould: the Invisible Menace *from Amazon UK.*

The air you breathe

Whether you are ill or just feeling under par, increasing the oxygen levels in your body will make you feel better. And improving the quality of the air you breathe is equally important.

Oxygen keeps your body working and your mind thinking. You can live without food for three weeks or more and without water for three to five days, but after approximately three minutes without air, you're unlikely to survive. Almost all the systems and activities of your body need oxygen to work properly, and around 90 per cent of your energy comes from oxygen too.

Today, there is less than half the amount of oxygen in the air we breathe than there was a century ago.[19] In 1900, air oxygen levels were 32 per cent. Today, oxygen levels all over the world are considerably reduced: as low as 15 per cent in the UK and 10 per cent in Tokyo. There has been a huge increase in air pollution levels, and an equal rise in tiredness and ill health. Most people know that around 60 per cent of the human body's weight is water, but did you know that as much as 65 per cent of that water is oxygen?[20] You can only top up the oxygen that your body needs by breathing.[21]

We breathe in and out an incredible 23,000 times every day. Most of the air we breathe is stale indoor air. Double-glazing and central heating means that the air in our homes often contains higher levels of pollutants than the air outside. The paint on your walls, the chipboard in your kitchen and even the fire-retardant sprays on that new sofa all give off invisible gases that can affect your health. The average UK adult spends around 80 per cent of their time indoors, which is estimated to be up to 10 times more polluted than outdoors – even allowing for traffic fumes.[22]

Cancer is now generally accepted to be a result of a lack of oxygen reaching the cells,[23] but low oxygen levels are also a factor behind the rise of many other diseases. Without oxygen, cells get weak and become targets for attack by the bacteria and viruses that multiply happily in an oxygen-depleted environment. Cells stop being able to repair themselves, break down toxins or do any of the jobs they are meant to properly. The brain and heart struggle too.

AIR QUALITY TEST

 Home

> The Atmotube (atmotube.com) is an inexpensive portable air pollution monitor that checks the quality of the air you breathe. It measures humidity, temperature, VOCs (volatile organic compounds) and harmful gases so you can make sure you and your family breathe healthy air.
>
> Alternatively, try the Office Air Check kit (homeaircheck. co.uk), which checks for mould, tobacco, formaldehyde and most major VOCs in the air around you. Along with an in-depth report, you are also given suggestions for improving the air quality.

Action plan

→ **Buy a pot plant or several:** Not only do plants look pretty but they are also an inexpensive way to clean up the air in your home. A NASA study found that specific varieties successfully neutralized the chemicals from household products, paints and furniture.[24] Spider plants, weeping figs, Boston ferns, aloe vera or a peace lily – take your pick.

→ **Get some air:** Opening your windows as often as possible is a natural way to filter the air and can be one of the most effective ways of assisting your lungs to dissipate the build-up.

→ **Invest in a Dyson Pure Cool™ air filter:** This removes 99.95 per cent of particles as small as 0.1 microns in the air inside your home. Not an inexpensive solution, but one that will last you a lifetime.

→ **Upgrade your vacuum cleaner:** Switch your normal vacuum for one with a HEPA (High Efficiency Particulate Air) filter and you'll remove around 99.7 per cent of the dust particles that can cause lung irritation. The filter also reduces lead concentrations and levels of fire-retardants, and removes pollens, dust mites and pet hair – all of which can overload your immune system and leave you with allergies and skin problems.

→ **Air safety:** Levels of NO2 (nitrogen dioxide) are 2.5 times higher inside the car than out. In fact, car drivers can be exposed to higher levels of air pollution inside their vehicle than on the pavement, suggesting that walking or cycling could be healthier. If you spend a lot of time in your car, then consider investing in an air purifier with a HEPA filter to eliminate smells, bacteria, pollen and dust along with air pollutants. Airbubbl is currently creating the first car filter that thoroughly cleans up the nitrogen dioxide levels inside your car (airbubbl.com).

➡ **Invest in an air ionizer for your home:** Placing an ionizer in your home can help to re-energize your home, and so reduce stress, anger and depression, and improve mood; they are inexpensive and simply plug in. Negative ions – the same molecules naturally found in waterfalls, rivers and by the sea – increase your ability to absorb oxygen and speed up its delivery to the cells and the tissues.

➡ **Avoid heavy traffic:** Air pollution comes mainly from road traffic, so take the back streets and avoid major busy roads when walking to the shops or to school.

➡ **Supplement:** Cellfood is a nutritional supplement combining minerals, enzymes and amino acids. A few drops in water or juice each day has been scientifically proven to oxygenate your body effectively. Chlorella and blue-green algae do the same. Oxy E is a liquid that contains seawater minerals, dissolved oxygen, plant-based amino acids and plant-based enzymes that oxygenate your cells, and also destroys free radicals. OxyTech is a magnesium and oxygen capsule that gently cleanses your colon, working through the gut walls to flood your body with oxygen (dulwichhealth.co.uk).

➡ **Oxygenize your diet:** Eating raw green food and a diet heavy in vegetables alkalizes your blood, releasing carbon dioxide and toxins and building oxygen levels naturally.

➡ **Breathe pure oxygen:** Medical centres offer hyperbaric oxygen treatments that let you breathe 100 per cent pure oxygen at higher than atmospheric pressure in an enclosed chamber. Some of the health claims made for this have been discredited, but it has been shown to reduce symptoms of a wide range of problems.[25] The same treatment used to help deep-sea divers recover from 'the bends', hyperbaric oxygen treatment forces oxygen deep into the body, where it is absorbed by your blood, liver, brain and all your cells and tissues, where it helps them repair and renew.

→ **Exercise:** Aerobic exercise several times a week is a powerful way to oxygenate your blood.

→ **Breathe:** Learning to breathe properly can improve your health better than most alternatives. Breathing deeply fills the bloodstream with oxygen and boots up your brain.

TOP TIP

The Buteyko breathing method was developed in the 1950s by Ukrainian doctor, Konstantin Buteyko, and is used worldwide today to overcome asthma and other breathing disorders.[26] Dr Buteyko taught patients to breathe through their nose rather than their mouth. He noticed that sick people only use their upper chest area to inhale air. This causes reduced levels of oxygen in the cells, as too much air is taken in with each breath, constricting the blood vessels. He found that 12 quiet breaths a minute, from the diaphragm and through the nose, was the most effective way to breathe, normalizing the volume of the breath, so that the tissues and organs of the body were better oxygenated.

Conclusion

Stay on Track

'The body is always talking to us, if we would only take the time to listen.'

LOUISE HAY

The trickiest part of any recovery programme is now. When you are in the grip of illness or a life-threatening disease, it is easier to make the choice to do whatever is necessary to help yourself. When you get better and daily life resumes as normal, it is all too easy simply to return to old patterns and habits.

Make a commitment to yourself to stay on track. Write an appointment with yourself in your diary now, once a month or every two months, to spend 10 minutes assessing your wellbeing.

Health checklist

There are also things it is sensible to do on a daily basis and others to keep an eye on from time to time, or even only once a year. Here is a quick checklist of things to put in place:

Diet

Design a diet that works for your body and your particular health issues alongside some simple guidelines that apply universally:

- Start the day with a glass of hot water with lemon or apple cider vinegar, then drink warm lemon and ginger water throughout the day.

- Drink a green juice every day.

- Eat more superfoods.

- Eat your food calmly and chew it well. Try to eat more in the morning and progressively less at each meal as the day progresses.

- Eat 50 per cent raw foods.

- Avoid eating too late in the evening.

- Take a daily multimineral and vitamin and any others that you know your body needs additional help with. Vitamin D3 with vitamin K2 should be taken daily.

- Drink at least 1.5 litres (3 pints) of pure filtered water a day.

- Add some blue-green algae in your diet to increase your energy and boost your immune system.[1]

- Boost your brain with fish oils, as they are important for blood pressure and immune system function.[2]

TOP TIP

In case you struggle with the idea of fish oil, Udo's Choice is an alternative blend of oils that has a balanced ratio of omega-3 and -6. It is gluten-free, organic and vegetarian. Krill oil, made from miniscule crustaceans, is one of the best sources of omega-3.

Exercise

Make sure you exercise and that it makes you happy – whether it's dance, walking, yoga or the gym. Find what works for you and try to do it three times a week. If it's close to where you live, you will probably find it easier to incorporate into your daily routine.

Watch your stress levels

There have been many studies on meditation showing it can help boost wellbeing – body and mind.[3-5] Start with five minutes' practice daily and build to about 15 minutes.

Get out in the sunshine

Get out in the sun daily, whatever the time of year. Sunshine is living energy and in healthy amounts supports all the body's systems, providing vitamins (particularly vitamin D), minerals and proteins, and affecting enzymes, hormones and many other things that contribute to health.

Sleep more

Make sure you are getting at least seven hours' sleep a night. The hours before 11 p.m. are the most valuable in health terms, so try to go to bed early once in a while.[6]

Cleanse

Get rid of the toxins that build up from everyday living. A steam bath or far-infrared sauna aids the removal of toxins from the body, and destroys bacteria and viruses. Have a bath once or twice a week with detoxifying Epsom salts to help remove heavy metals and other toxins via the skin and sweat. Daily dry skin brushing before you shower stimulates the lymphatic system to move the toxins out of your system. Do a parasite cleanse a couple of times a year to clear your gut.

Take a probiotic

Take a probiotic daily for six months or so to boost your beneficial intestinal flora.

Run the physical tests

Use the ones that work best for you once a year. Rebalance yourself according to any changes in results. For a full-body scan with 38 different tests in the space of an hour, book in with Dr John Ogden (see vitalityscreening.com for more information).

Laugh a lot

Ever since Norman Cousins cured himself from cancer by laughing and wrote a book to tell the world about it,[7] laughter has been taken seriously as a way to restore health. It can reduce blood pressure and stress levels, stimulate the heart and relieve muscle pain, all whilst increasing the good endorphins that reduce levels of pain and increase feelings of happiness in the body. Laughing relaxes and rejuvenates, and also stimulates the thymus. The stronger a person's sense of humour, the more resistant their immune system is to the effects of stress.

Update your relationships

Monitor who you spend regular time with every now and again, as sometimes we still hang out with people just because we've known them for 40 years. You will have changed in that time and so have they – and you may not even like them now. Remember that people are either like radiators, and warm and comfort you, or drains that leave you low and even depressed when you spend time with them. If you feel like someone is draining your energy, be aware. Spend less time with them or cut the relationship entirely if you can.

Write a list of the 10 people you spend the most time with and divide them into radiators or drains. Hopefully you will have many more friends under the radiator section, but if your drain list is full, then consider carefully if these friendships need to be re-evaluated.

Clear your clutter

At least once a year, block out some time to clear the clutter in your home and life to allow space for new things to come in. The difference it makes to the space you live in is palpable. Remember that your home is an extension of yourself. Fill it with things that make you happy.

TOP TIP

Research shows that clutter can decrease your productivity by up to 77 per cent; 68 per cent of people studied felt back in control of their lives once they had got rid of all their muddle.[8]

Commit to changing whatever needs changing

Review this one frequently. Don't put it off for another day. You could change your mind, your behaviour, your job, your home, your country – all things are possible. Many people get frozen in fear at the thought of all the changes they can see are necessary. A step at a time is all that is needed, and change works well as a slow and considered process. Imagine a captain steering a ship – a 10-degree movement of the wheel will still move the ship in a different direction.

Creating a healthy, happy life

There are few simple things that you can start doing right away that will increase your levels of wellbeing.

Don't waste time

Time is the most valuable thing we have and yet we so often waste it. Make sure you set time aside for yourself on a daily basis. Do something every single day that gives you pleasure. Look at how you spend your day and if you don't like it, change it. Give yourself a moment of space – to think, to read, to dream.

> ### TOP TIP
>
> *Do something kind for someone else too – it helps you as much as them, because it triggers the release of dopamine, as well as those happy-making endorphins, and oxytocin, which gives a sense of inner peace and calms stress levels in your body.[9] Write it in your diary – make it a date!*

Make room for those who matter

When we get busy with the minor things in life – paying bills, pulling out the weeds in the garden, cleaning the cupboards or washing and ironing – and add them to the bigger things we have to do – working and getting from A to B – the deepest and most important thing, your relationship with the people in your life who matter, sometimes gets side-lined. How long is it since you sat down and listened to what is going on in their lives and thoughts? How long is it since you had a long telephone call with an old friend, without being interrupted by the need to get on with your list?

Actively and consciously put time into your relationships. People often take the time to pay their respects by driving miles to a funeral – how much more valuable to the person who died to have had the time to spend with you when they were alive instead.

Slow down and pay attention

Don't miss out on life. When you're rushing from one place to another, running to do the endless things you've convinced yourself you need to do, you risk missing the things that make life worth living: the sunset; the flowers that have just bloomed, the children laughing or the smile of the old lady next door. Don't fill your life and get so busy that you miss the beginnings of things going wrong either. Don't be the person who missed the joy!

Communicate clearly – say 'no' if you want to

Often, we just presume that someone knows when we are angry or when we need help with something. But just because something is in your head, does not make it clearly visible to other people. Say it out loud – ask for help or let them know how you are feeling. Misunderstandings and mistakes can be avoided if people just talk. Many people want to please and often agree to do things that they don't really want to. Change this habit – practise saying no. You will be amazed how it will change your life!

Don't make others wrong so you can be right

Give up that there is anything wrong. Have you noticed how people are always complaining – about the weather, about the government, about just about everything? Be aware of the stories you tell yourself. The story we make up to blame someone else is usually in order to make ourselves right and to justify ourselves somehow. Stop doing it. Change your pattern and you will notice that things in your life, and the way people relate to you, also change – for the better. When you give off a different feeling, different things attract to you.

Change your reaction to stress

If something is 'getting' to you, find a way to 'change your mind' or change the situation. Don't just endure it. If you are sitting stationary in a traffic jam with your blood pressure rising, instead of railing about the waste of time and feeling powerless, use the experience as an unexpected gift and listen to an audio book or make some calls on your phone. Practice mindfulness and be thankful for the opportunity!

TOP TIP

It takes an average of 20 minutes to calm down after an emotionally driven reaction. So, take your time before you respond or you may make a decision you later regret.

Make a conscious choice to be happy

Do happy things and hang out with happy people. When you focus on the positive, you draw positive things to you. Do things that give you joy. Try to arrange at least one meeting a week with friends who strengthen you.

TOP TIPS

- *Control your addiction (because, don't kid yourself, that's what it is!) to your smartphone. Continually glancing at the screen whilst pretending to be focused on whatever you are meant to be doing is just not possible. Not only does it remove you from the moment, but it also sends a message to the person you are with that they are of less importance to you than your screen. Make a resolution to reduce your dependency – even if the best you can do is to put it away while you are eating with someone or in the middle of a conversation.*

• *The jury is still out on the safety of mobile phones, but to be on the safe side, protect your brain from any electromagnetic radiation by fixing a tiny GIA Cell Guard™ on the back of your phone – and on your computer too. Said to be 96 per cent effective, it is the only patented phone protection product on the market (see giawellness.com).*

Remove judgement

Does the critical voice inside you spend its time commenting nastily on everyone around you? 'Look at that terrible dress.' 'Goodness, he's ugly.' Imagine how much lighter you will feel if you put down all the baggage you've been carrying for someone else. Aim for nothing less than the death of that old habit. Remember:

• Walk a little way in other people's shoes and you will understand a lot more about them.

• Focus on the good in people, not the bad. Your world will change.

Don't make other people's stuff your business. Remember the phrase 'It's not my circus' and apply it to anything negative that comes your way. You are responsible for yourself before anyone else. Don't take on responsibility for everyone around you... even if it's done from love rather than guilt. Every bad decision has consequences for your health.

Be grateful

Begin your day with thanks for all the good things and people in your life by listing five things that you are grateful for. Really feel the emotion in your heart and spread the feeling throughout your body. People who are grateful have been shown to increase their happiness levels by 25 per cent.[10] Keep a gratitude diary and look back over it regularly.

How hard was it for you to find those five things? Appreciate everything that you take for granted. Every night before you go to bed, write down the things that have happened that day that make you grateful.

Going forwards

Put steps in place now for the months ahead that will remind you where you want to be with your health. Wear a fitness tracker on your wrist, book an annual blood test in advance, sign up to a membership at the gym, or book in for dance classes or healthy cooking demonstrations.

You may have successfully used this book to clear some of your current health issues, but others are likely to come your way from time to time. Work, relationships, money issues and health problems are on-going difficulties likely to rear their ugly heads in your life on occasion. If you stay in tune with yourself, you will pick up any signs and signals of stress well before any overload starts to build up. Deal with issues immediately to prevent your immune system from starting to struggle. Remember that the body always whispers before it shouts.

Keep listening and stay well.

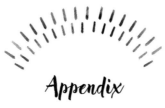

Appendix

Vitamins and Minerals

Vitamins		
Vitamin	Health benefits	Sources
A (beta carotene; derived from plant sources)	Antioxidant. Promotes skin health and liver function	Carrots, sweet potatoes, spinach, kale, broccoli, pumpkins, leafy greens, squash, watercress, papaya, cantaloupe melons
A (retinol; derived from animal products)	Antioxidant. Needed for eye health. Protects against respiratory infections. Promotes growth and healthy bones, teeth and gums. Vital for thyroid and hormone health. Protects against vitamin C depletion	Egg yolks and full-fat dairy products (especially butter), oily fish, fish liver oil (check for pollution), calves' liver, chicken thighs, venison, game, beef
B1 (thiamine)	Carbohydrate digestion and energy. Used by the nervous system and for cardiovascular health and mental health. Essential for thyroid (energy and body temperature) and adrenal glands (stress)	Fish (trout, salmon, tuna, mackerel), pork, seeds (sunflower, chia), nuts (pistachio, macadamia), edamame beans, peas, green beans, asparagus

Vitamins (continued)		
Vitamin	Health benefits	Sources
B2 (riboflavin)	Promotes healthy hair, skin and nails. Helps skin healing – sore mouths, lips and gums. Vital for energy production, stress management and pH balance. Colours the urine yellow. Reduces free radicals.	Leafy greens, spinach, mushrooms, broccoli, wild salmon, cottage cheese, watercress, almonds, eggs, beef liver, lamb, milk
B3 (niacin)	Vital for sex hormones, thyroid hormone, insulin, cortisone and GTF (glucose tolerance factor – blood glucose regulation). Helps promote healthy nervous system and mental health; also, fat metabolism, circulation and reducing cholesterol. High doses may cause flushing, so effective for stress headaches and migraine	Wheatgerm, wholegrains, brewer's yeast, avocados, cauliflower, dates, figs, eggs, chicken, lamb, turkey, tuna, peanuts, brown rice, liver, sweet potatoes, lentils, corn, mushrooms
B5 (pantothenic acid)	Converts fats and carbohydrates into energy. Needed to create antibodies supporting immune response and promotes wound healing. Vital for adrenal glands, sex hormone balance and joint function (effective in reducing symptoms of rheumatoid arthritis), Lowers cholesterol and triglycerides	Oatmeal, buckwheat, pecans, lentils, mushrooms, watercress, alfalfa, broccoli, cauliflower, avocados, eggs, strawberries, chicken liver, salmon, corn
B6 (pyridoxine)	Vital for fat metabolism. Needed to absorb B12 as well as magnesium and zinc. Vital for HCl (stomach acid) to enable protein digestion and make haemoglobin, amino acids and neurotransmitters. Essential for hormone balance and synthesis.	Chicken and turkey breast, grass-fed beef, salmon, tuna, pistachio nuts, avocados, sunflower seeds, chickpeas, bananas, walnuts, brown rice

Vitamins		
Vitamin	**Health benefits**	**Sources**
B6 (pyridoxine) (continued)	Vital for production of serotonin, melatonin and dopamine. May prevent kidney stones. May help decrease epileptic seizures. Protects against diabetic neuropathy as well as gestational diabetes	
B7 (biotin)	Helps body utilize carbohydrates, fats and proteins. Essential for healthy skin, scalp and hair. Enhances mood and energy. Prevents anaemia, nausea and hair loss. Destroyed by antibiotics, fried foods and excess intake of egg white	Brown rice, corn, tree nuts, egg yolks, cherries, almonds, carrots, peas, seeds, brewer's yeast, oatmeal, oysters, herring, green leafy vegetables, cauliflower, salmon, papaya, avocados, sweet potatoes
B9 (folic acid)	Regulates homocysteine (as B12). Essential for fertility and foetal development; also, antibody formation. Protects against parasites and food poisoning. Effective against restless legs syndrome with magnesium. Highly effective in reducing digestive disorders	Dark leafy greens (notably spinach), apricots, carrots, beans, bananas, cauliflower, asparagus, kidney beans, rye, wheatgerm, peanuts, avocados, wholegrains, squashes, pumpkins, broccoli, citrus fruits, lentils
B12 (cobalamin)	Essential for energy and helps blood carry oxygen. Regulates homocysteine. Enhances brain function – concentration, memory and mood. Vital for healthy DNA and RNA and red blood cell formation. Promotes healthy sperm count and motility	Meat, oysters, poultry, sardines, fish, shellfish, cottage cheese and eggs. Main vegetarian sources: kelp and jaggery (natural sugar alternative)

Vitamins (continued)		
Vitamin	**Health benefits**	**Sources**
C	Immune system builder: antiviral, antibacterial and enhances white blood cell formation. Reduces histamine secretion and allergy response. Effective for wound healing, healthy skin, bones, cartilage, muscle, gums, blood vessels and veins. Beneficial for heart, good blood pressure and regulating cholesterol. Also for adrenal health (stress recovery and hormone balance) and enhances iron absorption	Strawberries, citrus fruits, papaya, cabbages, cauliflower, cherries, broccoli, sweet and white potatoes, oranges, lemons, red peppers, parsley, kale, watercress, watermelon, blackcurrants, kiwis, broccoli
D	Vitamin D3 is the most important form for bone health and is both a hormone and a vitamin. Sunlight is the best source. Recent research identifies vitamin D as a powerful anti-cancer nutrient and antioxidant; also helps autoimmune disorders. Best known for stimulating calcium absorption (with magnesium). Low oestrogen, oestrogen blockers (tamoxifen) and magnesium deficiency affect vitamin D metabolism. Take a vitamin D3 supplement that also contains K2. Vitamin A taken at the same time will speed absorption.	Sunlight, cold water fish (mackerel, sardines, salmon, herring, cod), dark leafy greens, egg yolks, cottage cheese and butter. Synthetic vitamin D is often added to foods – cereals and bread – absorption can be weak

Vitamins		
Vitamin	**Health benefits**	**Sources**
E	Vital for sex hormones and sex drive. Potent antioxidant protects cell membranes, helps prevent scarring, acts as an anticoagulant and protects the thymus gland. Supplementation is useful for cardiovascular health, hormone imbalances, skin problems, inflammation, arthritis. Vitamin E will enhance vitamin A, B12, omega-3 essential fatty acids and selenium. D-alpha-tocopherol is the most effective form	Vegetable oils (pure, cold-pressed, unrefined), almonds, seeds, wholegrains, asparagus, avocados, berries, glossy leafy greens – such as watercress, spinach, tomatoes, sweet potatoes, fresh fish, organic eggs
K	Good for soft arteries and hard bones. Needed in combination with vitamin D3. Vitamin D enhances calcium absorption, but K2 sends the calcium to the bones rather than elsewhere in the body.	Broccoli, parsley, watercress, asparagus, Brussels sprouts, green beans, peas, carrots

Minerals		
Mineral	**Health benefits**	**Sources**
Calcium	Builds bones and teeth and used for blood clotting. Regulates heart beat and nerve transmission. May enhance iron absorption	Plant foods are less acidic sources of calcium than dairy: Brewer's yeast, kelp, kale, parsley, turnip tops, artichokes, green leafy veg (except spinach), almonds, dried figs, sunflower seeds, dried apricots, raisins, Brazil nuts, walnuts, chickpeas, raspberries, olives, watercress

Minerals (continued)		
Mineral	Health benefits	Sources
Chromium	Regulates insulin and blood glucose balance. Helps protein uptake. Can help reduce high LDL cholesterol and stabilizes blood sugar, reducing food cravings	Brewer's yeast, organic wholewheat, rye, potatoes, oysters, apples, pears, parsnips, cornmeal, bananas, organic eggs, beans, blueberries, carrots, mussels, oats, prunes, Brazil nuts
Iron	Important for red blood cell formation and energy production. Supports thyroid and helps metabolize B vitamins. Aids transportation of carbon dioxide from tissues to the lungs. Deficiency most common in pregnancy and those with heavy menstruation	Kelp, Brewer's yeast, wheat, pumpkin, spirulina, sunflower and sesame seeds, millet, parsley, clams, almonds, pistachios, prunes, raisins, Brazil nuts, dates, lentils, peas, beans, cherries, apricots, chicken, pork, tuna, beef liver, grass-fed beef, dark chocolate
Magnesium	Magnesium relaxes muscle pain and cramps and helps flexibility. Regulates calcium and energy production, and strengthens bones and teeth. Magnesium and vitamin B6 prevent kidney stones (and reoccurrence). Helps nervousness, hyperactivity and depression. Low magnesium levels associated with PMS, cramps, migraine, insomnia, stress, osteoporosis, arrhythmias, poor appetite and fatigue	Almonds, Brazil nuts, cashew nuts, avocados, wheatgerm, brewer's yeast, wholewheat flour, quinoa, buckwheat, spinach, kelp, seaweed, brown rice, figs, dried apricots, prunes, shrimps, edamame beans, white beans, French beans, peanuts, pecans, dark chocolate

Minerals		
Mineral	**Health benefits**	**Sources**
Manganese	Helps grow healthy bones, cartilage, nerves and tissue. Reduces inflammation and speeds up cellular repair from strains and sprains. Used by thyroid gland. Essential for digestion and enhances HDL cholesterol levels. Supports balance and coordination, as well as fertility. Good for brain and stabilizes blood sugar. Excess use of antacids, calcium, zinc and copper will inhibit manganese absorption	Pecans, Brazil nuts, almonds, rye, buckwheat, oats, walnuts, spinach, raisins, rhubarb, pineapples, raspberries, blackberries, black tea (leaves rather than teabags), carrots, egg yolks, beetroot, lettuce
Molybdenum	A component in several enzymes – especially alcohol detoxification, uric acid formation and sulphur metabolism. Molybdenum deficiency may be a cause of sulphite sensitivities (headache, nausea, shortness of breath)	Lentils, cauliflower, peas, spinach, brown rice, garlic, oats, rye, barley, onions, coconut, corn, pork, lamb, kidney beans, almonds, cashew nuts, soya beans, tofu, cheese, yoghurt, eggs
Phosphorous	Helps build strong bones and teeth. Enhances release of energy from food. Maintains pH balance. High doses can deplete calcium (phosphoric acid in fizzy drinks)	Lean red meat, fresh fish, poultry, brown rice, wholegrains, oats, nuts, seeds, buckwheat
Potassium	Helps nutrients move in and out of cells. Energy production, cardiovascular health (especially blood pressure), kidney and adrenal function, blood glucose regulation, water balance and distribution. Regulates pH levels	Avocados, molasses, watercress, celery, parsley, potatoes and sweet potatoes, greens, squashes, dried apricots, bananas, peaches, oranges, cod, salmon, chicken, coconuts, spinach

Minerals		
Mineral	**Health benefits**	**Sources**
Selenium	Supports immune system. Works with vitamin E to prevent free radical damage to cells. Low levels are associated with cancer, cardiovascular disease, inflammation, cataracts and excess levels of heavy metals (lead, cadmium, aluminium, mercury)	Brazil nuts, wholewheat, oats, barley, garlic, brown rice, organic tomatoes, fresh fish, shellfish, turnips, broccoli, walnuts, eggs, grass-fed beef, turkey, beef liver, chicken
Sulphur	Used by the body to make amino acids and proteins; keeps immune system and cells healthy. Taken as MSM controls pain and helps reduce inflammation. Without enough sulphur in the body, healing cannot take place. Can't be stored in the body and lack of it contributes to ageing and disease	Rocket, coconuts, cruciferous veggies (bok choy, broccoli, cabbages, cauliflower, horseradish, kale, kohlrabi, mustard leaves, radishes, turnips, watercress), dairy products (except butter), dried fruits, eggs, garlic, nuts, onions
Zinc	Essential for protein metabolism, growth, cell repair, enzyme production. Helps hormone balance, fertility, sex drive and blood glucose regulation. Excellent antistressor. Reduces hair loss and good for healthy skin, scalp and nails. Helps mental health (depression, anxiety, panic attacks, ADD/ADHD, concentration, memory and mood). Excellent results for preventing/reducing Alzheimer's and Wilson's disease. Enhances smell and taste acuity	Oysters, pumpkin seeds, sesame seeds, ginger root, pecans, Brazil nuts, organic wholewheat, rye, oats, oatmeal, lamb, almonds, buckwheat, peas, parsley, dark chocolate, garlic, chickpeas

References

Introduction: Why Settle for Poor Health?

1. Justice, B. *Who Gets Sick?* (Houston: Peak, 2000): 63
2. Passarino, G. *et al.* 'Human longevity: genetics or lifestyle? It takes two to tango', *Immun Ageing*, 2016; 13(1): 12

Chapter 1: The Heart: Your Life Force

1. http://www.who.int/mediacentre/factsheets/fs317/en/ [accessed 30 January 2018]
2. http://www.strokeassociation.org/STROKEORG/LifeAfterStroke/ HealthyLivingAfterStroke/Healthy-Living-After-Stroke_UCM_308568_ SubHomePage.jsp [accessed 30 January 2018]
3. https://www.medicinenet.com/stress_and_heart_disease/article.htm# heart_disease_and_stress_introduction [accessed 30 January 2018]
4. https://edition.cnn.com/2015/09/18/health/how-to-lower-blood-pressure-tips/index.html [accessed 30 January 2018]
5. https://www.nhs.uk/conditions/high-blood-pressure-hypertension/ prevention/ [accessed 30 January 2018]
6. https://www.nhs.uk/Livewell/Goodfood/Pages/saltaspx [accessed 30 January 2018]
7. https://www.ncbi.nlm.nih.gov/pmc/articles/PMC2682928/ [accessed 30 January 2018]
8. https://www.nutraingredients-usa.com/Article/2013/05/30/More-magnesium-may-slash-heart-disease-risk-by-30-Harvard-meta-analysis [accessed 30 January 2018]
9. Din, N. *et al.* 'Omega 3 fats and cardiovascular disease', *BMJ*, 2004; 328; 30–5
10. Hodgson, J, *et al.* 'Coenzyme Q10 improves blood pressure and glycaemic control: a controlled trial in subjects with type 2 diabetes', *Eur J Clin Nutr*, 2002; 56; 1137–42

11. https://www.ncbi.nlm.nih.gov/pubmed/28625322 [accessed 30 January 2018]

12. Susalit, E, *et al.* 'Olive (Olea Europaea) leaf extract effective in patients with stage-1 hypertension: comparison with captopril', *Phytomedicine*, 2011; 18(4): 251–8 doi: 101016/jphymed201008016; Epub Oct 30 2010

13. https://www.sciencedirect.com/science/article/pii/S2213177915008355 [accessed 30 January 2018]

14. https://www.nhs.uk/conditions/low-blood-pressure-hypotension/ [accessed 30 January 2018]

15. https://www.nhs.uk/conditions/vitamin-b12-or-folate-deficiency-anaemia/ [accessed 30 January 2018]

16. https://www.naturalmedicinejournal.com/journal/2012-03/siberian-ginseng-review-literature [accessed 6 February 2018]

17. https://lifespa.com/much-licorice-safe-blood-pressure-whole-licorice-vs-licorice-dgl/ [accessed 30 January 2018]

18. Manchanda, S. *et al.* 'Yoga and Meditation in Cardiovascular Disease', *Clinical Research in Cardiology*, 2014; 103(9): 675–80

19. Van Wormer, A. *et al.* 'The effects of acupuncture on cardiac arrhythmias: Literature Review,' *Heart Lung*, 2008; 37(6): 425–31

20. Michaud, G. *et al.* 'Relationship between serum potassium concentration and risk of recurrent ventricular tachycardia or ventricular fibrillation', *J Cardiovasc Electrophysiol*, 2001; 12(10): 1109–12

21. Kristensen, M. L. *et al.* 'The effect of statins on average survival in randomised trials, an analysis of end point postponement' BMI Open, Vol 5, Issue 9, 2014

22. Malhotra, A., *et al.* 'Saturated fat does not clog the arteries: coronary heart disease is a chronic inflammatory condition, the risk of which can be effectively reduced from healthy lifestyle interventions', *BJSM*, 2017 Aug; 51(15):1111–1112; doi:10.1136/bjsports-2016-097285

23. Ramsden, C.E. *et al.* 'Re-evaluation of the traditional diet-heart hypothesis: analysis of recovered data from Minnesota coronary experiment 1968–73', *BMJ* 2016; 353:i1246. doi: 10.1136/bmj.i1246

24. Ravnskov, U. *et al.* 'Lack of an association or an inverse association between low-densitylipoprotein cholesterol and mortality in the elderly: a systematic review', *BMJ Open* 2016; 6:e010401 doi: 10.1136/bmjopen-2015-010401

25. Rothberg, M.B. 'Coronary artery disease as clogged pipes: a misconceptual model', *Circ Cardiovasc Qual Outcomes*, 2013; 6:129–32; doi: 10.1161/circoutcomes.112/967778

26. Deichmann, R. *et al.* 'Coenzyme Q10 and statin-induced mitochondrial dysfunction', *Ochsner J*, 2010; 10(1): 16–21

27. Lamperti, C. *et al.* 'Muscle coenzyme Q10 level in statin-related myopathy', *Arch Neurol*, 2005; 62(11): 1709–12

28. https://www.healthline.com/nutrition/niacin-benefits [accessed 7 February 2018]

29. Stephens, N. *et al.* Randomised controlled trial of vitamin E in patients with coronary disease: Cambridge Heart anti-oxidant study', *Lancet*, 1996; 347(9004): 781–6

30. Stampfer, M. *et al.* 'Vitamin E consumption and the risk of coronary disease in women', *N Engl J Med*, 1993; 328: 1444–9

31. Von Schacky, C. *et al.* 'Cardiovascular benefits of omega-3 fatty acids', *Cardiovascular Research* Vol 73, Issue 2, 15 Jan 2007; 310–315

32. 'Low-dose aspirin vs vitamin e in cardiovascular disease' Am Fam Physician 2001 Aug 15; 64(4): 661–665

33. Carruthers, M. and Taggart, P. 'Vagotonicity of violence; biochemical and cardiac responses to violent films and television programmes', *BMJ*, 1973; 3(5876): 384–9

34. Kelly, J. and Sabate, J. 'Nuts and coronary heart disease: an epidemiological perspective', *Br J Nutr*, 2006; 96(2): S61–7

35. Rizos, C. *et al.* 'Effects of thyroid dysfunction on lipid profile', *Open Cardiovasc Med J*, 2011; 5; 76–83

Chapter 2: The Lungs: Your Breathing System

1. Shergis, J. *et al.* 'Herbal Medicine for adults with asthma: a systematic review', *J Asthma*, 2016; 53(6): 650–9

2. Trompette, A. *et al.* 'Gut microbiota metabolism of dietary fibre influences allergic airway disease and hematopoiesis', *Nat Med*, 2014; 20; 159–66

Chapter 3: The Stomach: Your Food Processor

1. https://www.healthline.com/nutrition/11-proven-ways-to-reduce-bloating#section11 [accessed 7 February 2018]

2. Britton, E. and McLaughlin, J. 'Ageing and acid reflux', *Proceedings of the Nutrition Society*, 2013; 72(1): 173–7

3. Iwai, W. *et al.* 'Gastric hypochlorhydria is associated with an exacerbation of dyspeptic symptoms in female patients', *Am J Gastroenterol*, 2013; 48(2): 214–21

4. Suarez, F. *et al.* 'Pancreatic supplements reduce symptomatic response of healthy subjects to a high fat meal', *Dig Dis Sci*, 1999; 44(7): 1317–21

5. Turpie, A. *et al.* Clinical trial of deglycyrrhizinate liquorice in gastric ulcer', *Gut*, 1969; 10; 299–303

Chapter 4: The Small Intestine: Your Food Blender

1. Foster, J. and McVey Neufeld, K. 'Gut-brain axis: how the microbiome influences anxiety and depression', *Trends in Neurosciences*, 2013; 36(5): 305–12

2. https://www.ncbi.nlm.nih.gov/books/NBK2486/ [accessed 30 January 2018]

3. https://www.ncbi.nlm.nih.gov/pmc/articles/PMC3152488/ [accessed 30 January 2018]

4. https://www.ncbi.nlm.nih.gov/pmc/articles/PMC3779803/ [accessed 30 January 2018]

5. Ley, R. *et al.* 'Microbial ecology: human gut microbes associated with obesity', *Nature*, 2006; 444: 1022–3

6. https://www.health.harvard.edu/blog/can-probiotics-help-treat-depression-anxiety-2017072612085 [accessed 30 January 2018]

7. Bezkorovainy, A. 'Probiotics: determinants of survival and growth in the gut', *Am J Clin Nutr*, 2001; 73(2): 399S–405S

8. Doron, S. *et al.* 'Lactobacillus GG: Bacteriology and Clinical Applications', *Gastroenterology Clinics*, 2005; 34(3): 483–98

9. https://www.ncbi.nlm.nih.gov/pmc/articles/PMC1774300/ [accessed 30 January 2018]

10. Messaoudi, M. *et al.* 'Assessment of psychotropic-like properties of a probiotic formulation (Lactobacillus helveticus R0052 and Bifidobacterium longum R0175) in rats and human subjects', *Br J Nutr*, 2011; 105(5): 755–64

11. Amara, A. and Shibl, A. 'Role of Probiotics in health improvement, infection control and disease treatment and management', *Saudi Pharmaceutical Journal*, 2015; 23(2): 107–14

12. http://www.bbc.co.uk/news/health-38800977 [accessed 14 February 2018]

13. Stiles, J. *et al.* 'The inhibition of candida albicans', *Oregano Journal of Applied Nutrition*, 1995; 47; 96–101

14. Yurdagul, Z. *et al.* 'The differential diagnosis of food intolerance', *Dtsch Arztebl Int*, 2009; 106(21): 359–70

15. www.ncbi.nlm.nih.gov/pubmed/9222036 [accessed 12 February 2018]

16. Liu, W. *et al.* 'Mechanisms of the bactericidal activity of low amperage electric current (DC)', *J Antimicrob Chemother*, 1997; 39(6): 687–95

Chapter 5: The Large Intestine: Your Food Compactor

1. https://www.cancer.org/latest-news/world-health-organization-says-processed-meat-causes-cancer.html [accessed 30 January 2018]

2. https://www.ncbi.nlm.nih.gov/pmc/articles/PMC2743456/ [accessed 30 January 2018]

3. Donovan, M. *et al.* 'Mediterranean Diet: Prevention of Colorectal cancer', *Front Nutr*, 2017; 4: 59

4. https://www.ncbi.nlm.nih.gov/pmc/articles/PMC4977816/ [accessed 30 January 2018]

5. Jung, L. *et al.* 'Fecal microbiota transplantation: a review of emerging indications beyond relapsing clostridium difficile toxin colitis', *Gastroenterol Hepatol*, 2015; 11(1): 24–32

6. https://www.webmd.com/digestive-disorders/poop-chart-bristol-stool-scale [accessed 30 January 2018]

7. Sanjoaquin, M. *et al.* 'Nutrition and lifestyle in relation to bowel movement frequency: A cross-sectional study of 20,630 men and women in EPIC', *Oxford Public Health Nutrition*, 2004; 7(1): 77–83

Chapter 6: The Pancreas: Your Blood Sugar Control

1. https://www.hsph.harvard.edu/news/press-releases/red-meat-type-2-diabetes/ [accessed 30 January 2018]
2. Robbins, T. and Harrelson, W. 'Simply Raw: Reversing Diabetes in 30 Days', 2009; https://www.fmtv.com/watch/simply-raw [accessed 30 January 2018]
3. Cousens, G. *There is a Cure for Diabetes* (North Atlantic Books, 2013)
4. Hsia, S. *et al.* 'Effect of Pancreas Tonic (an ayurvedic herbal supplement) in type 2 diabetes mellitus', *Metabolism*, 2004; 53(9): 1166–73

Chapter 7: The Liver: Your Detox Factory

1. Hamed, M. *et al.* 'Effects of black seed oil on resolution of hepato-renal toxicity induced by bromobenzene in rats', *European Review for Medical and Pharmaceutical Sciences*, 2013; 17(5): 569–81
2. https://www.livestrong.com/article/545154-elevated-liver-enzymes-fatigue/ [accessed 16 February 2018]

Chapter 8: The Gallbladder: Your Bile Producer

1. https://www.drdavidwilliams.com/importance-of-bile-acid [accessed 16 February 2018]
2. https://www.livestrong.com/article/337229-lipase-fat-digestion/ [accessed 16 February 2018]
3. http://naturalsociety.com/beet-borscht-a-natural-roto-rooter-for-the-congested-liver/ [accessed 16 February 2018]

Chapter 9: The Kidneys: Your Hydration Control

1. de Brito-Ashhurst, I. *et al.* 'Bicarbonate supplementation slows progression of CKD and improves nutritional status', *Journal of the American Society of Nephrology*, 2009; 20(9): 2075–84

Chapter 10: The Thymus: Your Immune System Manage

1. https://www.ncbi.nlm.nih.gov/pubmed/10202264 [accessed 30 January 2018]

Chapter 11: The Spleen: Your Immune System Support

1. https://news.osu.edu/news/2016/11/13/immunity-and-stress-sfn/ [accessed 30 January 2018]

Chapter 12: The Thyroid Gland: Your Hormone Production and Control

1. http://www.thyroiduk.org.uk/tuk/about_the_thyroid/hypothyroidism.html [accessed 30 July 2017]
2. https://www.ncbi.nlm.nih.gov/pubmed/22165143 [accessed 30 January 2018]

Chapter 13: The Adrenals: Your Stress Controllers

1. Cohen, S. *et al.* 'Chronic stress, glucocorticoid receptor resistance, inflammation and disease risk', *Proceedings of the National Academy of Sciences of the USA* 2012; 109(16): 5995–9

2. Allen, R. *et al.* 'Cinnamon use in type 2 diabetes: an updated systematic review and meta-analysis', *Ann Fam Med*, 2013; 11(5): 452–459

Chapter 14: The Blood: Your Vital Force

1. https://www.hindawi.com/journals/ecam/2014/642942/[accessed 30 January 2018]

2. Allen, R. *et al.* 'Cinnamon Use in Type 2 Diabetes: An updated Systematic Review and Meta-Analysis', *Ann Fam Med*, 2013; 11(5): 452–9

Chapter 16: The Skeleton: Your Structural Support

1. Patel, R. *et al.* 'Clinical evaluation of a phalangeal bone mineral density assessment system', *J Clin Densitom*, 2010; 13(3): 292–300

2. Garnero, P. *et al.* 'Increased bone turnover in late postmenopausal women is a major determinant of osteoporosis', *J Bone Miner Res*, 1996; 11(3): 337–49

3. Matheson, E. *et al.* 'The association between onion consumption and bone density in perimenopausal and postmenopausal non-Hispanic white women 50 years and older', *Menopause*, 2009; 16(4): 756–9

4. Gunn, C. *et al.* 'Increased intake of selected vegetables, herbs and fruit may reduce bone turnover in post-menopausal women', *Nutrients*, 2015; 7(4): 2499–517

5. Beasley, J. *et al.* 'Biomarker-calibrated protein intake and bone health in the Women's Health initiative clinical trials and observational study', *Am J Clin Nutr*, 2014; 99(4): 934–40

6. Klentrou, P. *et al.* 'Effects of exercise training with weighted vests on bone turnover and isokinetic strength in postmenopausal women', *J-Aging Phys Act*, 2007; 15(3): 287–99

7. Martyn-St James, M. and Carroll, S. 'Effects of different impact exercise modalities on bone mineral density in premenopausal women: a meta-analysis', *J Bone Miner Metab*, 2010; 28(3): 251–67

8. Moreira, L. *et al.* 'Physical exercise and osteoporosis: effects of different types of exercises on bone and physical function of postmenopausal women', *Arg Bras Endocrinol Metabol*, 2014; 58(5): 514–22

Chapter 17: Body Fat: Your Thermal Insulator

1. https://www.hopkinsmedicine.org/gim/core_resources/Patient%20Handouts/Handouts_May_2012/The%20Skinny%20on%20Visceral%20Fat.pdf [accessed 30 January 2018]

2. Report of a WHO expert consultation, 'Waist circumference and waist-hip ratio', Geneva, 8–11 December 2008

3.   https://www.precisionnutrition.com/thermogenic-foods [accessed 30 January 2018]

Chapter 18: The Last Pieces of the Jigsaw

1.   Vyas, B. and Le Quesne, S. *The pH Balance Diet: Restore Your Acid-Alkaline Levels to Eliminate Toxins and Lose Weight* (Berkeley, CA: Ulysses Press, 2007)

2.   Tobey, J. 'The question of acid and alkali forming foods', *Am. J. Public Health*, 1936; 26: 1113–6

3.   Schwalfenberg, G. 'The alkaline diet: is there evidence that an alkaline pH diet benefits health?', *J Environ Public Health*, 2012; ID 727630; doi: 101155/2012/727630 [accessed 6 June 2017]

4.   Young, R. and Young, S. *The pH Miracle for Weight Loss; Balance Your Body Chemistry, Achieve Your Ideal Weight* (Hachette, 2010)

5.   http://www.bstquarterly.com/Assets/downloads/BSTQ/Articles/BSTQ_2013-04_AR_Chronic-Inflammation-The-Cause-of-Disease.pdf [accessed 4 May 2017]

6.   Aggarwal, B. and Harikuman, K. 'Potential therapeutic effects of curcumin, the anti-inflammatory agent, against neurodegenerative, cardiovascular, pulmonary, metabolic, autoimmune and neoplastic diseases', *International Journal of Biochemistry and Cell Biology*, 2009; 41(1): 40–59

7.   White, B. and Judkins, D. 'Clinical inquiry: does turmeric relieve inflammatory conditions?' *J Fam Pract*, 2011; 60(3): 155–6

8.   Zarrouf, F. *et al.* 'Testosterone and depression: systemic review and meta-analysis', *J Psychiatr Pract*, 2009; 15(4): 289–305

9.   Sowers, M. *et al.* 'Testosterone concentrations in women aged 25–50 years: association with lifestyle, body composition and ovarian status', *Am J Epidemiol*, 2001; 153(3): 256–64

10. Panay, N. and Studd, J. 'The psychotherapeutic effects of estrogens', *Gynecol. Endocrinol*, 1998; 12(5): 5–9

11. Lee, J. *What Your Doctor May Not Tell You About Menopause* (Warner Books 2004)

12. https://www.ncbi.nlm.nih.gov/pmc/articles/PMC4082953/ [accessed 30 January 2018]

13. leBlanc, E. *et al.* 'Vitamin D and menopausal symptoms', *Menopause*, 2014; 21(11): 1197–1203

14. https://www.sciencedaily.com/releases/2007/08/070813185007.htm [accessed 6 February 2018]

15. http://tipsdiscover.com/health/anxiety-diet-address-pyroluria-low-levels-zinc-vitamin-b6/ [accessed 30 January 2018]

16. Woldenkirk, H. *et al.* 'Vitamin D and diabetes: its importance for beta cell and immune function', *Mol Cell Endocrinol*, 2011; 5: 106–20

17. Wacker, M. and Holick, M. 'Vitamin D – Effects on skeletal and extra-skeletal health and the need for supplementation', *Nutrients*, 2013; 5(1): 111–48

18. Welsh, J. 'Cellular and molecular effects of vitamin D on carcinogenesis', *Arch BiochemBiophys*, 2012; 523(1): 107–14

19. https://www.gov.uk/government/uploads/system/uploads/attachment_data/file/537616/SACN_Vitamin_D_and_Health_report.pdf [accessed 6 February 2018]

20. Heike, A. and Bischoff-Ferrari, M. *et al.* 'A pooled analysis of vitamin D dose requirements for fracture prevention', *New Engl J Med*, 2012; 367: 40–9

21. Vacek, J. *et al.* 'Vitamin D deficiency and supplementation and relation to cardiovascular health', *Am J Cardiol*, 2012; 109(3): 359–63

22. Bertone-Johnson, E. *et al.* 'Vitamin D intake from foods and supplements and depressive symptoms in a diverse population of older women', *Amer J Clin Nutr*, 2011; 94(4): 1104–12

23. Wolpin, B. *et al.* 'Plasma 25-hydroxyvitamin D and risk of pancreatic cancer', *Cancer Epidemiol Biomarkers Prev*, 2012; 21(1): 82–91

24. leBlanc, E. *et al.* 'Associations between 25-Hydroxyvitamin D and weight gain in elderly women', *J Womens Health*, 2012; 21(10): 1066–73

25. Kabadi, S. *et al.* 'Joint effects of obesity and vitamin D insufficiency on insulin resistance and type 2 diabetes: results from the NHANES 2001–2006 2012', *Diabetes Care*, 2012; 35(10): 2048–54

26. Terushkin, V. *et al.* 'Estimated equivalency of vitamin D production from natural sun exposure versus oral vitamin D supplementation across seasons at two US latitudes', *J AM Acad Dermatol*, 2010; 62(6): 929

27. Mulligan, G. and Licata, A. 'Taking vitamin D with the largest meal improves absorption and results in higher serum levels of 25-hydroxyvitamin D', *American Society for Bone and Mineral Research*, 2010; 25(4): 928–30

28. http://copperalliance.org.uk/docs/librariesprovider3/pub-183-impact-of-copper-on-human-health-pdf.pdf?Status=Master&sfvrsn=0 [accessed 7 February 2018]

29. https://metabolichealing.com/histamine-allergies-brain-gut-health/ [accessed 13 February 2018]

Chapter 19: Food Fundamentals

1. Taylor, R. *et al.* 'Primary care-led weight management for remission of type 2 diabetes: an open-label cluster-randomised trial', *Lancet*, 2017; 391(10120): 541–55

2. Howell, E. *Enzyme Nutrition* (Avery, 1995)

3. https://fcs-hes.ca.uky.edu/sites/fcs-hes.ca.uky.edu/files/fn-ssb.006.pdf [accessed 6 February 2018]

4. www.who.int/features/qa/cancer-red-meat/en/ [accessed 6 February 2018]

5. Bouvard, V. *et al.* 'Carcinogenicity of consumption of red and processed meat', *The Lancet Oncology*, 2015; (16): 1599–1600

6. Zhang, C. *et al.* 'Genetically modified foods: A critical review of their promise and problems', *Food Science and Human Wellness*, 2016; 5(3): 116–23

7. https://www.livestrong.com/article/198975-what-are-the-dangers-of-palm-oil/

8. https://www.ewg.org/release/apples-top-dirty-dozen-list-fifth-year-row#.Ws32yi_Mwkg [accessed 7 February 2018]

9. http://www.worldactiononsalt.com/less/how/other/index.html [accessed 7 February 2018]

10. Dasgupta, P. K. *et al.* 'Iodine nutrition: iodine content of iodized salt in the United States', Environ. Sci. Technol. 2008, January 9. 42 (4), pp 1315–1323 doi: 10.1021/es0719071

11. https://www.americanbluegreen.com/study.html [accessed 7 February 2018]

12. Hendel, B. and Ferreira, P. Water and Salt: The Essence of Life (Natural Resources Inc. 2001)

13. Xiao, C. 'Health effects of soy protein and isoflavones in humans,' Journal of Nutrition, 2008; 138(6):1244S–1249S.

14. Forsythe, W. 'Soy Protein, thyroid regulation and cholesterol metabolism, Journal of Nutrition, 1995; 125(3): 619S–623S

15. Messina, M. *et al.* 'Gaining insight into the health effects of soy but a long way still to go: commentary on the fourth International Symposium on the Role of Soy in Preventing and Treating Chronic Disease', Journal of Nutrition, 2002; 132(3): 547S–551S

16. Tovar, A. Navalta, J. *et al.* 'The effect of moderate consumption of non-nutritive sweeteners on glucose tolerance and body composition in rats', Appl Physiol Nutr Metab, 2017; 42 (11): 1225–7; doi: 10.1139/apnm-2017-0120

17. https://www.ncbi.nlm.nih.gov/pubmed/28394643 [accessed 7 February 2018]

18. Hsieh, M. Chan, P. *et al.* 'Efficacy and tolerability of oral stevioside in patients with mild essential hypertension: A two-year, randomized, placebo-controlled study', Clinical Therapy, 2003; 25(11): 2797–808

19. Taavoni, M. Ekbatani, B. *et al.* 'Effect of valerian on sleep quality in postmenopausal women: a randomised placebo-controlled clinical trial. Menopause, 2011; 18(9): 951–5

20. Udani, J. Singh, B. *et al.* 'Effects of Acai berry preparation on metabolic parameters in a health overweight population: a pilot study', Nutr J, 2011; 10: 45

21. Fauce, S. Jamieson, B. *et al.* 'Telomerase-based pharmacologic enhancement of antiviral function of human CD8+ T lymphocytes', J Immunol, 2008; 181(10): 7400–6

22. Singh, N. Bhall, M. *et al.* 'An overview on ashwagandha: a rejuvenator of Ayurveda', African Journal of Tradition, Complementary and Alternative Medicines, 2011; 8(5): 208–13

23. https://www.hindawi.com/journals/ecam/2015/297425/ [accessed 7 February 2018]

24. Nehlig, A. 'The neuroprotective effects of cocoa flavanol and its influence on cognitive performance', Br J Clin Pharmacol, 2013; 75(3): 716–27

25. https://www.hindawi.com/journals/bmri/2012/171956/ [accessed 7 February 2018]

26. https://www.hindawi.com/journals/ecam/2014/642942/ [accessed 7 February 2018]

27. Bucheli, P. et al. 'Goji Berry effects on macular characteristics and plasma antioxidant levels', Optom Vis Sci, 2011; 88(2), 257–62

28. https://www.ncbi.nlm.nih.gov/pmc/articles/PMC2855614/ [accessed 7 February 2018]

29. Girgih, A. et al. 'Reverse-phase HPLC separation of hemp seed (Cannabis sativa L.) protein hydrolysate produced peptide fractions with enhanced antioxidant capacity', Plant Foods Hum Nutr, 2013; 68(1): 39–46

30. Lee, M. et al. 'Maca (Lepidium meyenii) for treatment of menopausal symptoms: A systematic review', Maturitas, 2011; 70(3): 227–33

31. Gonzales, C. et al. 'Effects of different varieties of Maca on bone structure in ovariectomized rats', Forsch Komplementmed, 2010; 17(3): 137–43

32. http://www.foxnews.com/health/2013/01/23/healing-power-olive-leaf.html [accessed 7 February 2018]

33. http://www.oleaft.com/medical-evidence/ [accessed 7 February 2018]

34. Fleming, J. et al. 'Olea europaea leaf (Ph. Eur.) extract as well as several of its isolated phenolics inhibit the gout-related enzyme xanthine oxidase', Phytomedicine, 2011; 18(7): 561–6

35. Panossian, A. Wikman, G. Sarris, J. 'Rosenroot (Rholdiola rosea): Traditional use, chemical composition, pharmacology and clinical efficacy', Phytomedicine, 2010; 17: 481–93

36. http://www.macoc.fr/resources/The+Journal+of+the+American+Nutraceutical+Association+vol+5+spring+2002+Spiruline.pdf [accessed 7 February 2018]

37. Kuptniatsaikul, V. et al. 'Efficacy and safety of curcuma domestica extracts compared with Ibuprofen in patients with knee osteoarthritis: a multicenter study', Clin Interv Aging, March 2014; 9: 451–8

38. Dey, S. et al. 'Effect of Wheat grass juice in supportive care of terminally ill cancer patients – a tertiary cancer centre experience from India', J Clin On 2006; 24(18): 8634

39. MacWilliam, L. Comparative Guide to Nutritional Supplements (North Dimensions Publishing, 2007; 4th edition)

40. Belay, et al. 'Current knowledge on potential health benefits of spirulina', Journal of Applied Phycology, 1993; 5: 235–41

41. https://www.iatp.org/files/scarcity_of_micronutrients.pdf [accessed 17 June 2017]

42. https://www.energy-medicine.org/qxci.html [accessed 14 February 2018]

43. Klok, M. *et al.* 'The role of leptin and ghrelin in the regulation of food intake and body weight in humans: a review', Obesity Reviews, 2007; 8(1): 21–34

44. Hansen, T. *et al.* 'Weight loss increases circulating levels of ghrelin in human obesity', Clinical Endocrinology, 2002; 56(2): 203–6

45. Schmid, S. Hallschmid, M. *et al.* 'A single night of sleep deprivation increases ghrelin levels and feelings of hunger in normal weight healthy men', Journal of Sleep Research, 2008; 17(3): 331–4

46. Tanaka, M. *et al.* 'Habitual binge/purge behaviour influences circulating ghrelin levels in eating disorders', Journal of Psychiatric Research, 2003; 37(1): 17–22

Chapter 20: Water Works

1. https://water.usgs.gov/edu/propertyyou.html [accessed 11 May 2017]

2. Boschmann, M. *et al.* 'Water Drinking Induces Therogenesis through Osmosensitive Mechanisms', J Clin endocrinol Metab, 2007; 92(8): 3334–7

3. Boschman, M. *et al.* 'Water-induced thermogenesis', J Clin endocrinol Metab, 2003; 88(12): 6015–9

4. https://adaa.org/understanding-anxiety/related-illnesses/other-related-conditions/stress/physical-activity-reduces-st# [accessed 12 February 2018]

5. Armstrong, L. *et al.* 'Mild dehydration affects mood in healthy young women,' J Nutr, 2012; 142(2): 382–8

6. Ganio, M. *et al.* 'Mild dehydration impairs cognitive performance and mood of men', Br J Nutri, 2011; 106(10): 1535–43

7. Shireffs, S. *et al.* 'The effects of fluid restriction on hydration status and subjective feelings in man', Br J Nutri, 2004; 91(6): 951–8

8. http://jech.bmj.com/content/69/7/619.long [accessed 12 February 2018]

9. Hu, X. *et al.* 'Detection of poly-and perfluoroalkyl substances in us drinking water linked to industrial sites, military fire training areas and wastewater treatment plants', Environ Sci Techno, 2016; 3(10): 344–50

10. https://nywea.org/clearwaters/08-3-fall/05-EstrogenInWastewater.pdf [accessed 27 July 2017]

11. https://nyulangone.org/press-releases/yearly-exposure-to-chemicals-dangerous-to-hormone-function-burdens-americans-with-hundreds-of-billions-in-disease-costs [accessed Jan 2017]

12. Stephenson, C. and Flanagan, G. 'Synthesis of Novel Anionic Hydride Organosiloxane presenting biochemical properties', Int J Hydrog Energy, 2003; 28: 1243–50

13. Batmanghelidj, F. Your Body's Many Cries for Water: You are Not Sick, You are Thirsty (Tagman Press, 2007)

14. http://phisciences.co/research [accessed 14 February 2018]

15. Hye-Jin Lee and Myung-Hee Kamg. 'Effects of the magnetised water supplementation on blood glucose, lymphocyte DNA damage, antioxidant status, and lipid profiles in STZ-induced rats', Nutrition Research and Practice, 2013; 7(1): 34–42

16. Quickenden, T. *et al*. 'Effect of magnetic fields on the pH of water', Journal of Physical Chemistry, 1971; 75(18): 28930–1

17. Tovstoles, K. *et al*. 'The histologists of the S.M. Kirov Military Medical Academy – their contribution to practical medicine', Arkh Anat Gistol Embriol, 1991; 101(9–10): 5–18

18. http://www.rainlikewater.com/blog/2012/09/the-health-benefits-of-magnetic-water/ [accessed 12 February 2018]

Chapter 21 – Stand Tall: Fitness Facts

1. https://digital.nhs.uk/catalogue/PUB13648 [accessed 7 February 2018]

2. https://www.amssm.org/research-says-regular-exe-p-145.html [accessed 7 February 2018]

3. Scully, D. Kremer, J. Meade, M. *et al*. https://www.amssm.org/research-says-regular-exe-p-145.html 'Physical exercise and psychological well being: a critical review', British Journal of Sports Medicine, 1998; 32: 111–20

4. https://www.health.harvard.edu/press_releases/benefits-of-exercisereduces-stress-anxiety-and-helps-fight-depression [accessed 13 February 2018]

5. Yates, T. *et al*. 'Self-reported sitting time and markers of inflammation, insulin resistance and adiposity', American Journal of Preventive Medicine, 2012; 42(1): 1–7

6. O'Keefe, J. *et al*. 'Potential adverse cardiovascular effects from excessive endurance exercise', Mayo Clin Proc, 2012: 87(7): 704

7. Cresswell, D. *et al*. 'Affirmation of personal values buffers neuroendocrine and psychological stress responses', Psychological Science, 2005; 16(11) 846–51

8. www.hse.gov.uk/Statistics/causdis/musculoskeletal/msd.pdf [accessed Jan 2016]

9. DeokJu, K. *et al*. 'Effect of an exercise program for posture correction on musculoskeletal pain', Journal of Physical Therapy Science, 2015; 27(6): 1791–4

10. Carney, D. *et al*. 'Power posing: brief nonverbal displays affect neuroendocrine levels and risk tolerance', Psychological Science, 2010; 21(10): 155–7

11. Peper, E. *et al*. 'increase or decrease depression: how body postures influence your energy level', Biofeedback, 2012; 40(3): 125–30

Chapter 22 – Stress: The Hidden Menace

1. https://www.nimh.nih.gov/health/publications/stress/index.shtml [accessed Jan 2016]

2. Holford, P. *et al.* '100% Health Survey: A Comparison of the Health and Nutrition of Over 55,000 People in Britain (Holford & Associates, 2010)

3. Gonzalezs-Diaz, S. *et al.* 'Psychoneuroimmunoendocrinolgoy: clinical implications', World Allergy Organ Journal, 2017; 10(1): 19

4. Cohen, S. *et al.* 'Psychological stress and disease', JAMA, 2007; 298(14): 1685–7

5. Brown, R. and Gerbarg, P. 'Sudarsha Krya Yogic Breathing in the Treatment of Stress, Anxiety and Depression: Part 1', Journal of Alternative and Complementary Medicine, 2005; 11(1): 189–201

6. Hoge, E. *et al.* 'Randomized controlled trial of mindfulness meditation for generalized anxiety disorder: Effects on Anxiety and Stress Reactivity', J Clin Psychiatry, 2013; 74(8): 786–92

Chapter 23: Reboot Your Sleep

1. Morris, A. *et al.* 'Sleep quality and duration are associated with higher levels of inflammatory biomarkers: the META-Health Study,' Presented at the American Heart Association, 2010 Scientific Sessions, Chicago

2. Pines. A. 'Sleep duration and midlife women's health', Climacteric, 2017; 14:1–3; doi: 10.1080/13697137.2017.1335702 [accessed 30 July 2017]

3. https://www.ncbi.nlm.nih.gov/pubmed/28707143 [accessed 6 February 2018]

4. Wehrens, S. *et al.* 'Meal timing regulates the human circadian system', Curr Biol, 2017; 27(12): 1768–75

5. https://www.sciencedaily.com/releases/2013/10/131023183908.htm [accessed 14 February 2018]

6. Wood, B. *et al.* 'Light level and duration of exposure determine the impact of self-luminous tablets on melatonin suppression', Appl Ergon, 2013; 44(2): 237–40

7. Krauchi, K., *et al.* 'Thermoregulatory effects of melatonin in relation to sleepiness', Chronobiology International, 2006; 23(1&2): 475–84

8. Tipple, C. *et al.* 'A review of the physiological factors associated with alcohol hangover', Current Drug Abuse Reviews, 2016; 9(2): 93–8

9. Taavoni, M. *et al.* 'Effect of valerian on sleep quality in postmenopausal women: a randomised placebo-controlled clinical trial', Menopause, 2011; 18(9): 951–5

10. Montgomery, P. *et al.* 'Fatty acids and sleep in UK children: subjective and pilot objective sleep results from the DOLAB study – a randomized controlled trial', Journal of Sleep Research, 2014; 23(4): 364–88

11. Liu, A. *et al.* 'Tart cherry juice increases sleep time in older adults with insomnia. Journal of the Federation of American Societies for Experimental Biology, 2014; 28(1): supplement 830.9

12. https://www.ncbi.nlm.nih.gov/books/NBK11941/ [accessed 26 February 2017]

Chapter 24 – Environment Essentials

1. Woodruff, T. *et al*. 'Environmental Chemicals in Pregnant Women in the US: NHANES 2003–2004', Environmental Health Perspectives, 2011; 119(6): 878–85

2. Jyaratnam, J. 'Acute pesticide poisoning: a major global health problem', World Health Stat, 1990; Q 43: 139–44.

3. Calle, E. *et al*. 'Organochlorines and breast cancer risk', CA Cancer J Clin, 2002; 52: 301–9

4. https://www.maurerfoundation.org/bisphenol-a-bpa-the-breast-cancer-link/ [accessed 6 February 2018]

5. http://www.breastcancer.org/risk/factors/plastic [accessed 6 February 2018]

6. http://www.breastcanceruk.org.uk/reduce-your-risk/protect-your-family/ [accessed 6 February 2018]

7. Bouma, K. and Schakel, D. 'Migration of phthalates from PVC toys into saliva simulant by dynamic extraction', Food additives and Contaminants, 2010; 19(6): 602–10

8. Fischer, M. 'The toxic effects of formaldehyde and formalin', J Exp Med, 1905; 6(4–6): 487–518

9. Dinwiddie, M. *et al*. 'Recent evidence regarding triclosan and cancer risk', Int Journal of Environmental Research and Public Health, 2014; 11(2): 2209–17

10. Jurewicz, J. and Hanke, W. 'Exposure to phthalates: Reproductive outcome and children health. A review of epidemiological studies', Int Journal of Occupational Medicine and Environmental Health, 2011; 24(2): 115–41

11. https://cfpub.epa.gov/ncea/iris/iris_documents/documents/subst/0326_summary.pdf [accessed Jan 2016]

12. https://www.cancer.org/cancer/cancer-causes/teflon-and-perfluorooctanoic-acid-pfoa.html [accessed Jan 2016]

13. https://www.scientificamerican.com/article/should-people-be-concerned-about-parabens-in-beauty-products/ [accessed Jan 2016]

14. http://time.com/4229503/plastic-in-microwave-is-it-safe/ [accessed 7 February 2018]

15. Kondo, M. The Life-changing Magic of Tidying (Vermilion, 2014)

16. https://f1000research.com/articles/5-366/v1 [accessed Jan 2016]

17. https://www.sciencedaily.com/releases/2007/08/070813185007.htm [accessed Jan 2016]

18. Jaishankar, M. *et al*. 'Toxicity, mechanism and health effects of some heavy metals', Interdisciplinary Toxicology, 2014; 7(2), 60–72

19. https://www.theguardian.com/commentisfree/2008/aug/13/carbonemissions.climatechange [accessed Jan 2016]

20. https://askabiologist.asu.edu/explore/building-blocks-life [accessed 7 February 2018]

21. Vanderkooi, J. Your Inner Engine: An Introductory Course on Human

Metabolism (CreateSpace Independent Platform, 2014): Ch 10: Delivering Oxygen

22. Environmental Protection Agency, 'Factors Affecting Indoor Air Quality', 2016: 5–12

23. Warburg, O. 'The Metabolism of Tumours', Journal of General Physiology, 1927; 8(6): 519

24. https://ntrs.nasa.gov/search.jsp?R=19930072988 [accessed Jan 2016]

25. Grim, P. *et al.* 'Hyperbaric Oxygen Therapy', JAMA, 1990; 263(16), 2216–20

26. Bowler, S. *et al.* 'Buteyko breathing techniques in asthma: a blinded randomised trial', Medical Journal of Australia, 1998; 169: 575–8

Conclusion: Stay on Track

1. Belay, A. *et al.* 'Current knowledge on potential health benefits of spirulina', Journal of Applied Phycology, 1993; 5: 235–41

2. Geleijnse, J. *et al.* 'Blood pressure response to fish oil supplementation: metaregression analysis of randomized trials', Journal of Hypertension, 1979; 20(8): 1493–9

3. Farb, N. *et al.* 'Minding one's emotions: mindfulness training alters the neural expression of sadness', Emotion, 2010; 10: 25–33

4. Raes, F. *et al.* 'Mindfulness and reduced cognitive reactivity to sad mood: evidence from a correlational study and non-randomized waiting list controlled study', Behaviour Research and Therapy, 2009; 47: 623–7

5. Epel, E. *et al.* 'Can meditation slow rate of cellular aging? Cognitive stress, mindfulness and telomeres', Annals of the New York Academy of Sciences, 2009; 1172: 34–53

6. Donga E. *et al.* 'A single night of partial sleep deprivation induces insulin resistance in multiple metabolic pathways in healthy subjects', Journal of Clinical Endocrinology Metabolism, 2010; 96(6): 2963–8

7. Cousins, N. Anatomy of an Illness (WW Norton & Company, 1979)

8. http://news.officedepot.com/press-release/officemax-historical/national-survey-reveals-workplace-clutter-tarnishes-professional- [accessed 6 February 2018]

9. Emmons, R. and McCullough, M. 'Counting blessings versus burdens: an experimental investigation of gratitude and subjective well-being in daily life', J Pers Soc Psychol, 2001; 84(2): 377–89

10. http://sb.cc.stonybrook.edu/news/general/122111StephenPost.php [accessed 6 February 2018]

Index

E

eating
    and appetite 186–8
    avoiding drinking with meals
      177
    a balanced/diverse diet 69, 174
    chewing habits 37, 42, 244
    do's and don'ts 174–81
    falling asleep after 44
    late night avoidance 220, 244
    portion size 22, 42, 176
    and sleep 44, 220, 221
    see also food
echinacea 96
eczema 61
    and probiotics 51
EDTA chelation 233
eGFR (glomerular filtration rate) 91
eggs 254, 257, 260
    enzymes 40
    excess egg white destroying
      biotin 255
    yolk 253, 254, 255, 256, 258
electrolytes 89, 110, 115, 122
electromagnetic fields (EMFs)
    232
Emotional Freedom Technique
    (EFT) 92, 223
endorphins 160, 182, 214, 246, 248
enemas *see* colonics and enemas
energy
    and blood glucose 110
    boosts 108, 115, 124, 131, 147, 153,
      183
    depletion with sitting for long
      periods 205
    flow 95, 147, 149
    lack of 24, 43
    scanning 7–8
    of sunshine 245 *see also*
      sunlight
    TCM and the energy system
      99–100, 147–8 *see also*
      acupuncture
    white fat storage of 31, 137
environment 228–42
    air quality 32, 238–42
    clearing the clutter 231, 247
    heavy metals *see* heavy metals
    mould 234–8

pesticides 49, 83, 175, 191,
    227–8, 230, 232
pollution 32, 83, 239, 240–41
    and sleep hygiene 219–20
    and the thyroid 107–8
    the toxic home 228–32, 234–8
enzymes 39–42, 175
    aids 39–42, 57
    digestive 36, 39, 40–41, 42, 54,
      57, 73, 77, 151
    gallbladder-strengthening 87
    and the liver 81
    and molybdenum 259
    natural 40
    and sunshine 245
    systemic 41–2
    and zinc 260
eosinophils 122
Epsom salts 220, 245
ergonomic chairs 206
ERMI (Environmental Relative
    Mouldiness Index) 236
erythrocyte sedimentation rate
    (ESR) 122, 155–6
essential oils 136, 160, 214, 231
Ete plate 176
eucalyptus 34
exercise 72, 196–7, 245
    action plan 201–2
    aerobic 242
    and blood pressure 196
    to burn off fat 137
    cardiovascular 198
    and cholesterol 18
    core-strengthening 201, 206
    and digestion 196
    and emotional stress 214
    Fitness Blender 201
    and the heart 196, 197
      heart rate 26, 198, 200
    and hypertension 18–19
    lack of 16
    for lymph support 131
    machines 135
    and the menopause 160
    Pilates 204
    running 197
    and stress 197, 214
    and the thymus 96
    walking *see* walking

lungs 32–5
 measuring lung functions
 33–4
lymphatic system 129–32
 action plan to support 131–2
 lymph nodes 130, 131, 132
 lymphoedema 130–31
 manual lymphatic drainage
 massage 132
lymphocytes 122, 129

M

maca 161, 182, 214
mackerel 20, 30, 169, 256
magnesium 92, 93, 109, 114, 135,
 136, 152, 165, 170, 175, 193, 213,
 244, 258
 deficiency 20
 sulphate 220
magnetized water 194–5
maltase 40
manganese 128, 165, 175, 258–9
mannitol 56
Mapmygut.com 69
MCH (mean corpuscular
 haemoglobin) 120
McTimoney chiropractic 204
MCV (mean corpuscular volume)
 120
meal size 22, 42, 176
meat 175, 253, 254, 255, 259, 260
 lean 87
 and the liver 82
 parasites in 62
 processed 77, 135, 175
 red 65
 smoked 65
 undercooked 62
 white 29
 see also beef; lamb; pork
meditation 24, 92, 98, 245
 mindfulness 213
melatonin 218, 219, 221, 255
menopause 158–62
mercury 107, 191, 232, 233, 234
microbiome 47–50, 180
migraines 180, 208, 254, 258
milk enzymes 40
milk thistle 83, 99
mimosa pudica powder 63

mindfulness 213
 see also meditation
minerals 257–60
 for adrenal support 114
 for bone growth 135, 136
 deficiencies
 calcium 152
 and full body scans 184
 iodine 106–7, 116
 iron 61, 123
 magnesium 20, 152
 molybdenum 259
 potassium 152
 selenium 115, 260
 sodium 152
 zinc 162, 165
 for emotional stress 213
 hair mineral analysis test 107,
 169, 233
 heavy metals see heavy metals
 and the kidneys 92, 93
 for leaky gut 57
 loss in cooked foods 175
 for low histamine 170
 lowering colon cancer risk 65
 multiminerals 244
 for stabilizing blood sugar levels
 128
 in standard blood test results
 122
 and sunshine 245
 supplements
 iodine 106, 116
 magnesium 93, 109
 selenium 65, 109
 for thyroid support 109
 zinc 57, 109
 and the thyroid 105–6, 107,
 108
mirror test for inflammation 154
mobile phone addiction 250–51
molybdenum 259
monocytes 122
monosodium glutamate (MSG)
 156, 188
mould 234–8
moxibustion 99–100
MPV (mean platelet volume) 121
MSM 260
mullein 54

ABOUT THE AUTHOR

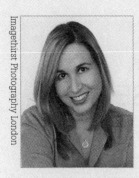

Sara Davenport is one of the UK's top health entrepreneur philanthropists and campaigners, and has been at the centre of the wellbeing sector for three decades.

Twenty years ago, driven by a conviction that despite improvements in cancer treatments, patients were feeling unsupported and disempowered, Sara sold everything she owned to fund the creation of the charity Breast Cancer Haven. It is now one of the UK's leading breast cancer charities, with six national centres in London, Hereford, Leeds, Worcester, Hampshire and Solihull.

Through her work with doctors, nutritionists and therapists, Sara has an unrivalled view of both traditional and complementary medicine. She travels the world to ensure she is up to date with the latest healing approaches in other countries, and her aim is to achieve health through non-invasive, inexpensive methods, working hand in hand with conventional medical treatments.

Sara founded and writes the blog ReBoot Health, which features articles covering a wide range of health issues and offers simple but effective natural solutions to a wide variety of problems. She discusses remedies that work and things that don't, all based on personal experience and years of research and study. Sara is on a mission to help everyone to learn about the basics of health, and provide the tools to help them take responsibility for their wellbeing and live a healthy, happy life.

www.reboothealth.co.uk
www.breastcancerhaven.org.uk

HAY HOUSE
Look within

Join the conversation about latest products,
events, exclusive offers and more.

f Hay House UK

🐦 @HayHouseUK

📷 @hayhouseuk

💜 healyourlife.com

We'd love to hear from you!